Contents

1 Working with text: Robots!

By the end of this unit you will:

→ understand how to use the shift key

→ learn how to change the colour, size and style of a word

→ know how to use pictures and words together

→ learn how to move text to the middle of the page

→ understand how to print your work.

In this unit you are going to make a guide to robots.

A robot is a machine that can do human things.

In real life robots can be used in many ways. For example, in factories to make cars or electronics. Some robots can be used to travel underwater!

In our imaginations robots can do almost anything!

Most robots are made up of three parts:

→ The 'controller'. This is a computer program that works like the brain.

→ Mechanical parts. These make the robot move.

→ Sensors. These tell the robot what is going on around it.

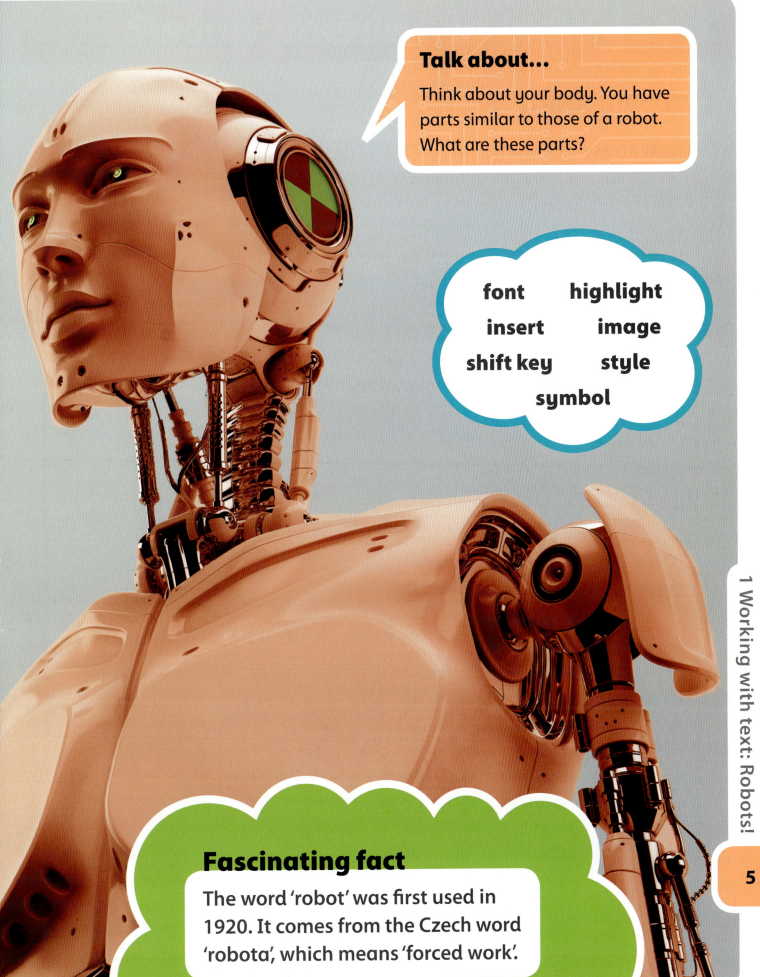

Talk about...

Think about your body. You have parts similar to those of a robot. What are these parts?

font   highlight
insert   image
shift key   style
symbol

Fascinating fact

The word 'robot' was first used in 1920. It comes from the Czech word 'robota', which means 'forced work'.

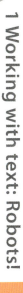

You will learn:

→ how to open and save a new file
→ about the keyboard and its functions
→ how to be courteous when using technology.

How to open a file

Do you remember how to open a new file?
Look at the toolbar.

1 Click on 'File.'

2 Click 'New.'

Can you find your way around the
keyboard? What do all these keys do?

1 The numbers.

2 The letters.

3 This is the backspace key.

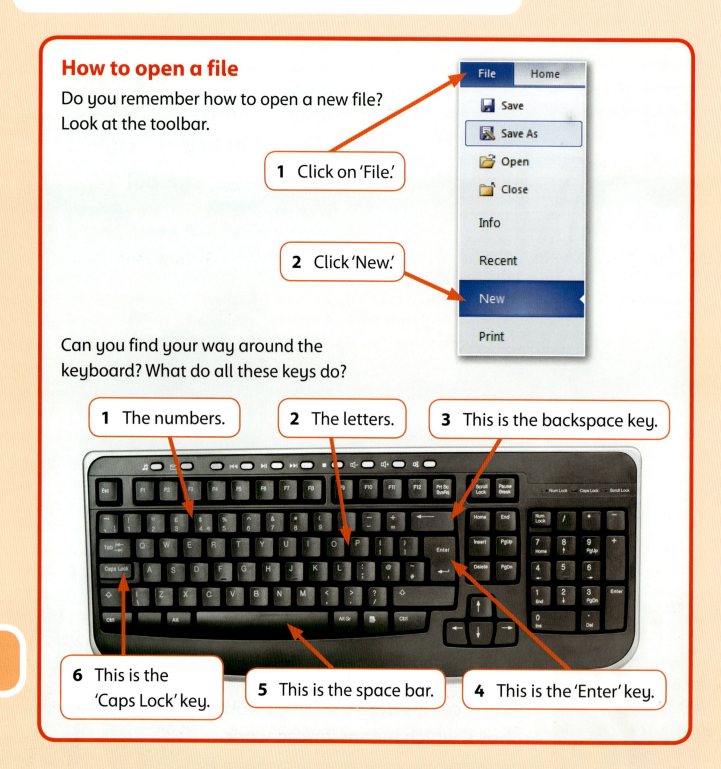

6 This is the 'Caps Lock' key.

5 This is the space bar.

4 This is the 'Enter' key.

How to save a file

Do you remember how to save your file? This is how to save your file.

1 Click 'File.' **2** Move the cursor to 'Save As.' **3** Click 'Save As.'

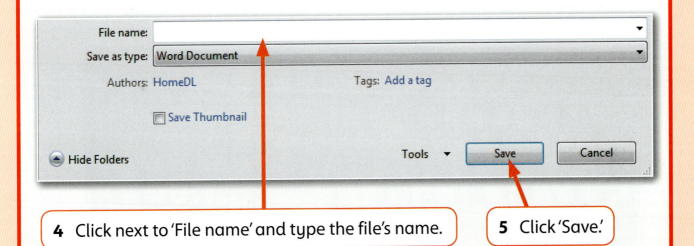

File name:	
Save as type:	Word Document
Authors:	HomeDL	Tags: Add a tag
	☐ Save Thumbnail

⊙ Hide Folders   Tools ▼   **Save**   Cancel

4 Click next to 'File name' and type the file's name.   **5** Click 'Save.'

Activity What do I know?

⊙ Look at the worksheet your teacher has given you.

1 Draw a smiley face if you feel confident to do the task.

2 Write a '?' if you are unsure.

3 Look at the instructions on page 6 and above. Try each of the tasks.

4 Now look at your worksheet again. Do you feel more confident about your skills? Draw smiley faces where you feel more confident.

Talk about...

If you had a robot, what jobs would you make it do?

If you have time...

Explain to a partner what courteous use of technology means.

You will learn:

→ how to use the shift key.

You already know many keys on the keyboard.

1 'Caps Lock'

2 The numbers.

3 The letters.

4 The backspace key.

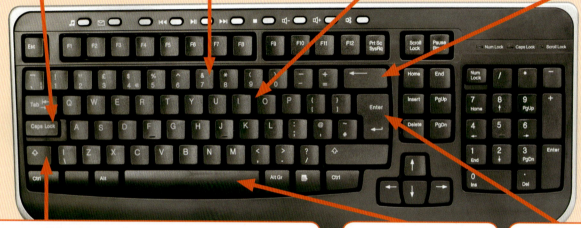

We are going to learn about the shift key.

6 The space bar.

5 The 'Enter' key.

We use the **shift key** to type the **symbols** at the top of a key. Symbols are the characters on the key.

How to use the shift key

Find the '1' key.

What do you see above the number '1'?

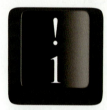

Use the shift key to type the '!'

Now find the '/' key. What do you see above the symbol '/'?

Use the shift key to type the '?'

To make these symbols appear you have to press down and hold the shift key, and press the key at the same time.

Activity Using the shift key

Open a new file.

1 Find the '1' key again.

2 Press and hold down the shift key.

3 Press '1'.

Lift your fingers off the keys.

What can you see on the screen?

4 Now try it with the '/' key.

 5 Now look at the symbols, letters and numbers your teacher has given you. Can you find them all?

Can you make a drawing of a robot using the symbols on the number keys to draw the body?

 If you have time...

Make a pattern using only symbols you can type using the shift key.
For example:

@@&*"@@&*"@@&*"@@&*"

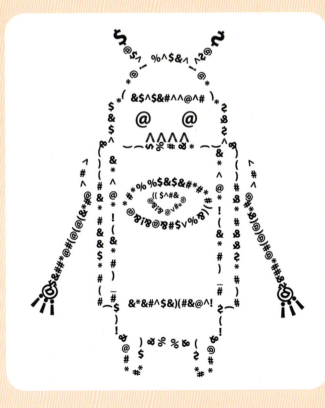

You will learn:

→ how to change the size of a word.

You already know how to change the colour of a word to make it look more interesting.

Making words bigger and smaller can make them look interesting too.

A bigger **font** size makes the text bigger.

This is font size 36.

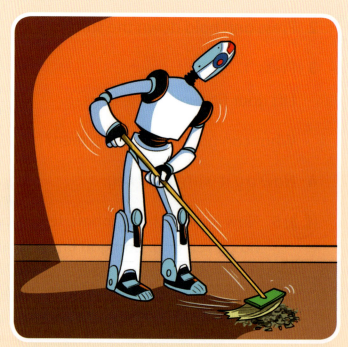

A smaller font size makes the text smaller.

This is font size 8.

Most text we use is font size 11 or 12.

How to make text bigger

Make the font size bigger or smaller by changing the font size number.

1 Click 'Home'.

2 This is the font size icon.

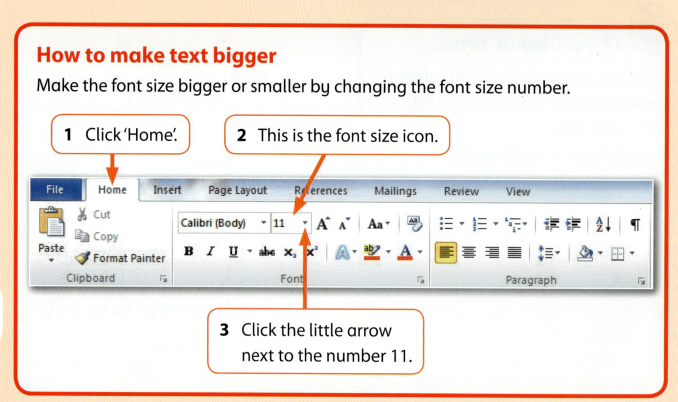

3 Click the little arrow next to the number 11.

Activity | Changing the size of a word

 Look at the text on the screen.

It is about robots.

1 Highlight a word you would like to be bigger.

You can do this by clicking on the front of the word, holding down the mouse button, and pulling or dragging the mouse along until the word is highlighted. Let go!

2 Look at the toolbar and click 'Home'.

3 Find the font size icon and arrow. Click the number '20'. Click back on your page.

Your word should be big.

4 Highlight the word again. Click back on your page.

5 Find the font size icon and arrow again. Click the number '8'.

Your word should be small.

Now type a sentence about your robot. Make one word big or small.

Talk about...

Imagine if you had a robot.

What would you make it do?

Would it do your cleaning?

Would it make you delicious food?

Would it be able to speak?

What would it look like?

 If you have time...

Type some more sentences about your robot for your robot guide.

You will learn:

➔ how to change the **style** of a word.

You already know how to change the colour and size of a word to make it look more interesting (see Student Book 2, Unit 1, lesson 5).

We can also change the way a word looks to make it look special.

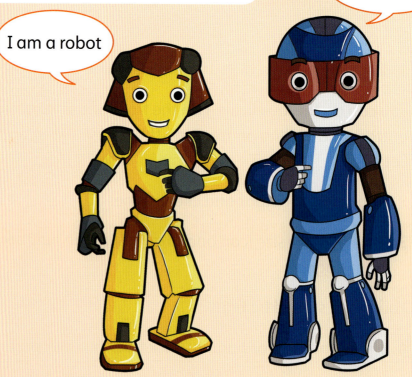

I am a robot

I am a robot

How to change the font style

Look at the words on the screen.

Highlight the word you would like to change.

Look at the 'Home' tab.

Choose and click on one of the font style names.

1 Click 'Home'.

2 This is the font style icon.

3 Click on this little arrow to see more font style names.

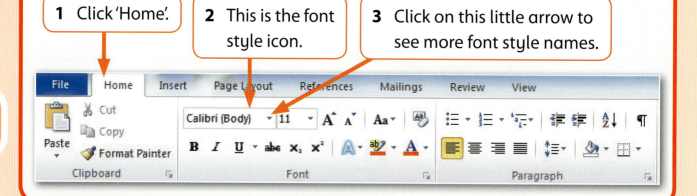

Activity Changing the style of a word

1 Open your file about your robot.

2 Add two more sentences to your text about your robot.

Here are some ideas:

→ What job does it do?

→ What is it made of?

→ Is it big or small?

→ Is it friendly?

3 Now follow the instructions on page 12 to change the style of three words in your text. Think carefully about which words you change.

 If you have time...

Which font style do you like best?
Why do you like that font?

You will learn:

→ how to put an **image** on your page.

Words together with pictures are easier to understand than words or pictures on their own.

You will need pictures as well as words for your guide to robots. We call putting a picture into a file '**inserting** an image'.

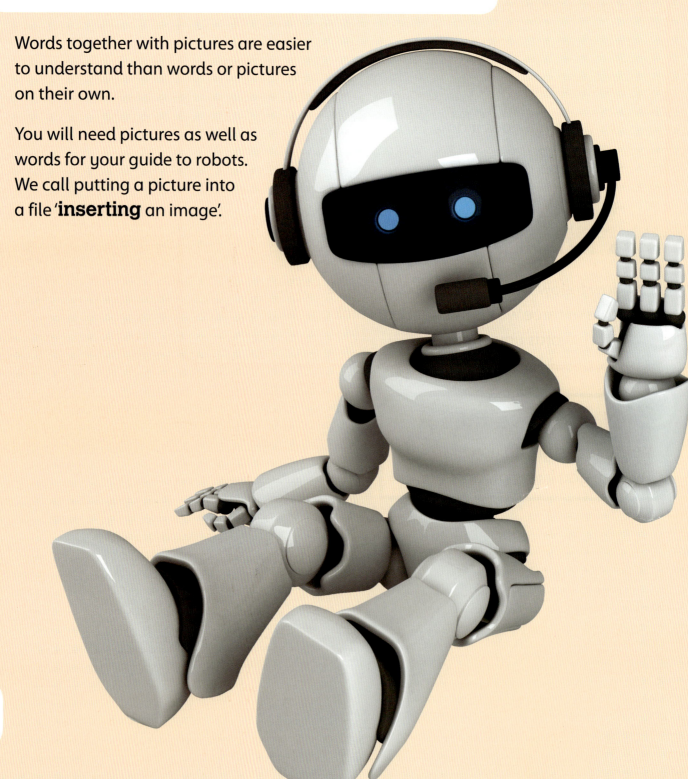

How to insert an image

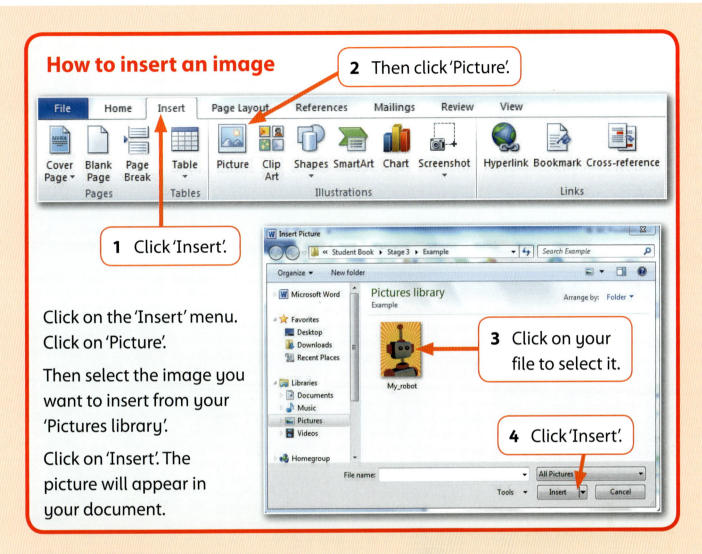

2 Then click 'Picture'.

1 Click 'Insert'.

Click on the 'Insert' menu. Click on 'Picture'.

Then select the image you want to insert from your 'Pictures library'.

Click on 'Insert'. The picture will appear in your document.

3 Click on your file to select it.

4 Click 'Insert'.

Activity | Insert an image

 1 Open your 'Guide to Robots' file.

2 Press the 'Enter' key two times after your sentences.

3 Look at the toolbar. Follow the instructions above.

4 Select the image you are guided to by your teacher.

Your picture should appear on the screen.

 Remember to save your file!

 If you have time...

You can make your picture bigger or smaller by moving your cursor to the corner of your image.

You will see your cursor change to a double arrow. Click and hold the mouse button. Move the mouse to make the image bigger or smaller.

You will learn:

➜ how to print a page.

Do you know what paper is made of?

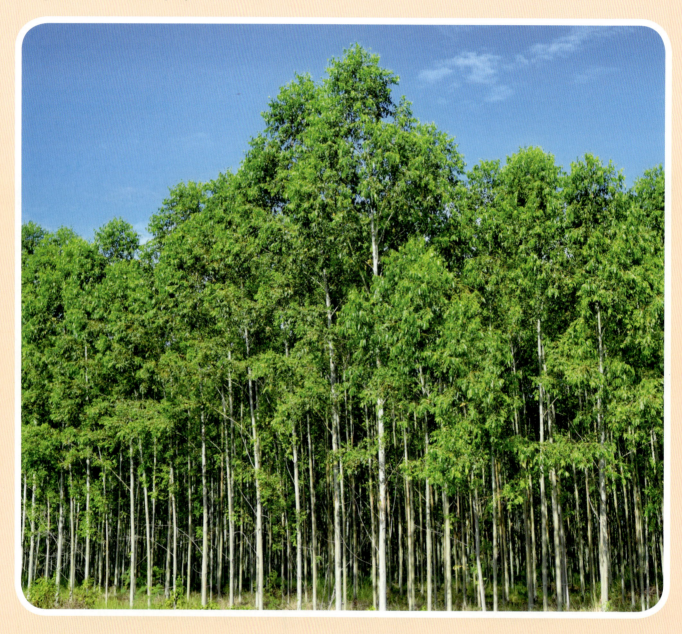

We try not to print too much because we do not want to waste paper.

Sometimes we do need to print our work so that we can share it with others.

Activity **Printing your work**

1 Open your 'Guide to Robots'. Look at the top of the page.

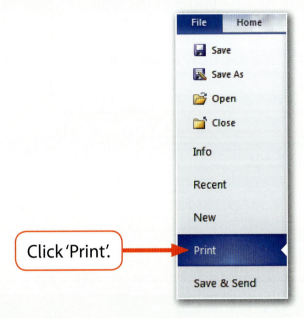

Click 'Print'.

2 Look for this icon and click on it.

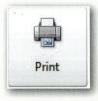

Talk about...

Share your work with someone else in the class. Let them share their work with you. Talk about:

➔ things you like about each other's work

➔ things you could do better next time.

What you have learned about working with text

You have learned how to use the shift key; how to change the colour, size and style of a word; how to use pictures and words together; how to move text to the middle of the page; and how to print your work.

The activities on this page will let you see how much you have learned.

1 Write down the names of these keys.

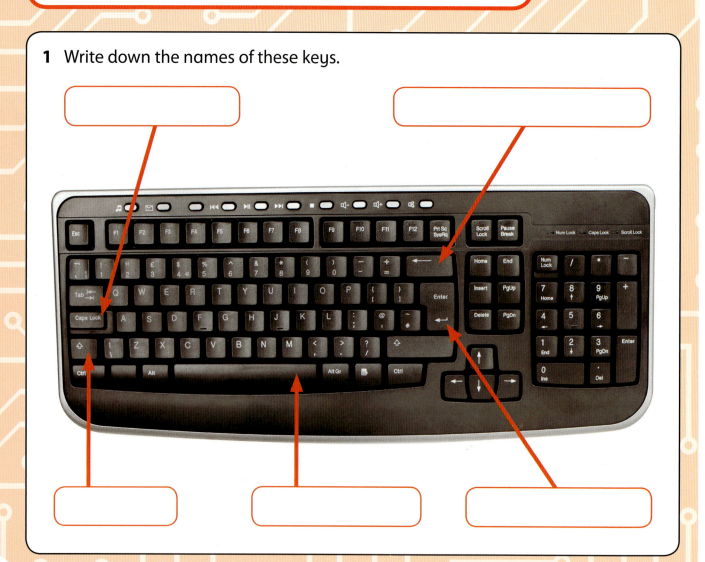

2 What do these words mean?

- font

_____

_____

- image

_____

_____

- insert

_____

_____

Activity Make a word look special

Type these words and then make them look special for your teacher.

Make this word big: robot.

Make this word small: sensors.

Make this word a colour: controller.

Make this word a different style: mechanical.

2 Multimedia: My robot presentation

By the end of this unit you will:

→ plan and make a slideshow

→ make slides with words and pictures

→ use animations in your slideshow to make a quiz

→ deliver your presentation to your classmates.

In this unit you are going to create a presentation to introduce your robot to your classmates.

A presentation is a way of sharing your ideas with a group of people. You can use a presentation program like *Microsoft PowerPoint* to make slides.

The slides will help your audience understand your presentation.

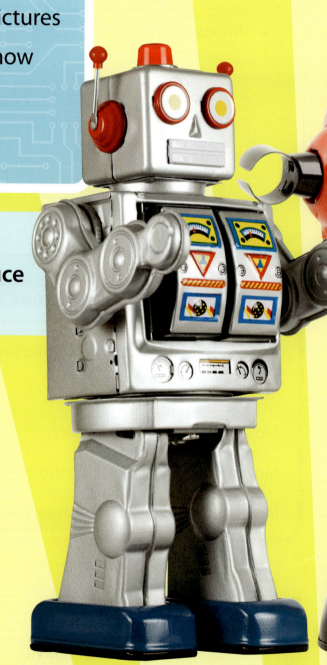

20

Activity   What is a presentation?

Write down all the things that make up a presentation.

Think of the people, the room and the equipment that might be included.

presentation
transition   callout
animation
import   slide

Fascinating fact

More than 30 million presentations are created around the world every day.

You will learn:

→ how to plan a presentation.

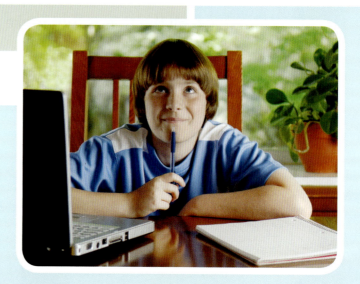

Planning a **presentation** is really important. A presentation is like a story. It should have three parts: a beginning, a middle and an end. You need to think carefully about what you want to say in each part.

How to plan your presentation

1 Think about what you need to say to help your audience understand the information in your presentation.

2 Think about how much time you have for your presentation. Make sure you don't use too many **slides**.

My Personal robot

Everything you need to know!

What I'm going to talk about

- My robot's name
- What he is like
- What he can do
- A quiz to test your memory

My robot Bod

- My robot is called Bod.
- He is green and yellow.
- He is friendly and kind.
- He always listens to me.

What my robot can do

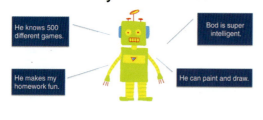

He knows 500 different games.

Bod is super intelligent.

He makes my homework fun.

He can paint and draw.

My robot quiz

- What is my robot's name?
  Bod
- What colours is he?
  Green and Yellow
- Is he kind or nasty?
  Kind
- How many games does he know?
  500

▲ About five slides are enough for a short presentation.

3 Think about the best way to present your information. You can use pictures as well as text.

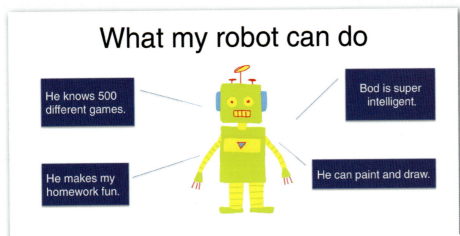

What my robot can do

He knows 500 different games.

Bod is super intelligent.

He makes my homework fun.

He can paint and draw.

4 Think about some ways to help your audience remember the things you say. You can:

→ add a summary at the end

→ ask some questions.

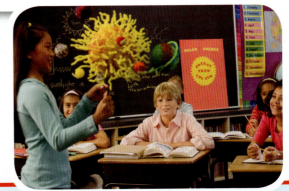

Activity | Plan your presentation

1 On a piece of paper, write down what you want to say about your robot. Choose the most interesting things about it, for example its name, what it looks like, and what it can do. Write down each thing on a separate line.

2 Now choose what order to present your information in. Write a number next to each bit of information. Number 1 will become your first slide.

3 Now decide what each slide will look like. Will it have text? Or a picture? Or both?

Talk about...

What makes a good title?

What makes a good introduction?

You will learn:

➔ how to choose a slide layout
➔ how to add text to a slide.

Start your presentation about your personal robot with a title and an introduction. These two slides will have text on them.

How to make a title slide

When you start a new presentation *MS PowerPoint* will give your first slide a special 'Title Slide' layout.

> You can change the font and the font size if you want to.

Click in each box on the slide to type your 'title' and 'subtitle'. You can put your name in the subtitle box.

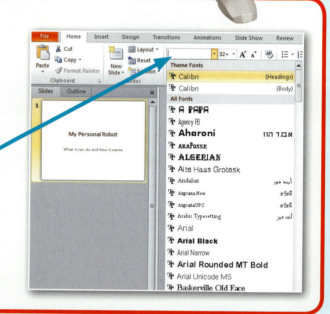

How to add an introduction slide

Click on the bottom of the 'New Slide' button to add a new slide for your introduction. Choose a 'Title and Content' layout from the drop-down menu.

This slide tells your audience what your presentation is about.

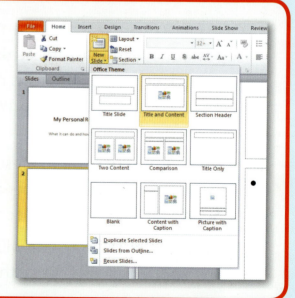

Put a heading in the top box and put your introduction in the bottom box.

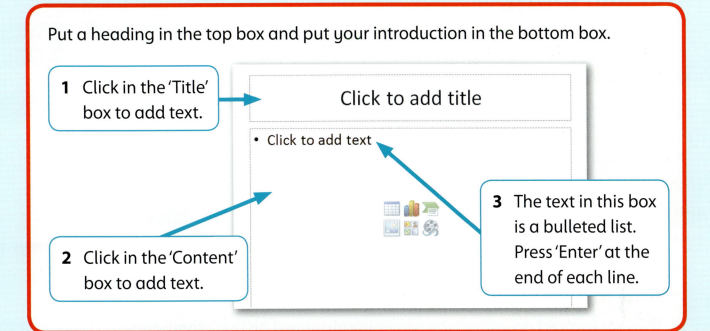

1 Click in the 'Title' box to add text.

Click to add title

• Click to add text

2 Click in the 'Content' box to add text.

3 The text in this box is a bulleted list. Press 'Enter' at the end of each line.

Activity | Create a new presentation

1 Open *Microsoft PowerPoint*.

2 On the first slide, add your presentation title and subtitle in the text boxes. You can use your name as a subtitle.

3 Add a new slide with a 'Title and Content' layout.

4 On the new slide, add a heading and your introduction text.

💭 Remember to look at your work from the last lesson so you know what your introduction should say.

🕐 If you have time...

Use the font menus to change the way your text looks. Find your favourite font.

💭 Remember, your presentation must be easy for your audience to read. Don't make the text too small!

You will learn:

→ how to add an image to your presentation
→ how to create a drawing using Shapes
→ how to add text to explain your picture.

To make your robot presentation more interesting you can put text and images together. You can add photos, drawings and charts to your slides.

My Mega Droid

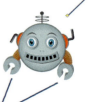

- This is my Mega Droid
- He is a personal robot that can fly
- He is powered by a computer brain
- He tidies my room and does my homework
- He is amazing!

A big computer brain to do my homework

Special hands to tidy my room

How to insert images on your slides

You can **import** an image you have already saved on your computer.

Images can be:

→ a drawing you made in another program, like *Microsoft Paint*
→ a photograph you have saved
→ a clip art image.
→ You can even make your own image using Shapes.

2 If you are using clip art, search for and select your image in the clip art window.

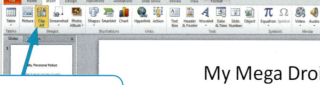

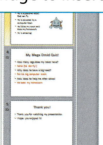

1 Click on a button to choose the type of image to insert.

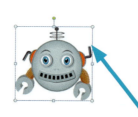

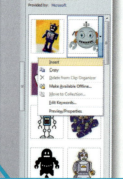

3 Move, resize and rotate the image with your mouse.

26

How to add text

You can add text in a separate box. This will make your slide look very neat.

Sometimes you might want to put your text closer to the image to help explain it. You can use a **callout** to do this.

1 Choose a 'Callout' shape from the 'Shapes' drop-down menu.

2 Click on the slide and drag the mouse to draw the shape. Move and resize the shape with the mouse.

3 Click in the shape and type your callout text.

4 Drag the yellow diamonds to move the lines.

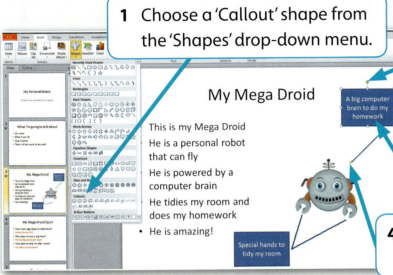

Activity   Create a new slide with an image

1 Open your *Microsoft PowerPoint* presentation about your robot.

2 Insert a new slide. Choose a slide layout that will give you space for text and an image.

3 Add an image to your slide.

4 Add the heading for your slide in the correct box.

5 Add your text in the correct box.

◀ Try using the 'Shapes' menu to draw a picture of your robot.

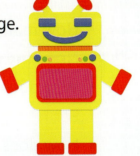

If you have time...

Add some callouts to your image to show the most interesting parts of your robot.

You will learn:

→ how to use animations in a presentation.

You can make your slides more exciting by adding movements to the text and images.

Each movement is called an **animation**.

You can also use animations to control when text and images appear on your slide.

In this lesson you are going to use animations to make a quiz for your audience.

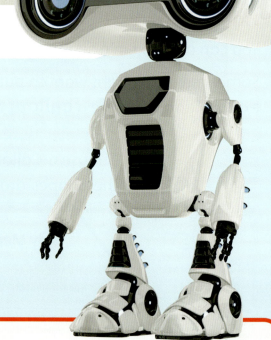

How to make a quiz with animations

Type some questions and answers on a slide.

Then use animations to make the answers appear later.

My Mega Dro...

- How many legs does my robot have?
- None (he can fly!)
- Why does he have a big head?
- For his big computer brain
- How does he help me after school?
- He does my homework

1 Choose a slide layout with space for some questions and answers. Type the questions and answers on separate lines.

3 Choose an animation from the menu.

2 Select and highlight each answer.

You can see a demonstration of how each animation will look. Choose your favourite one.

Check how your slide will look by going to the 'Slide Show' menu. Click on the 'From Current Slide' button.

Click the mouse button once to reveal each answer!

Talk about…

What kind of questions can you ask in your quiz?

Activity   Use animations to make a quiz

1 Open your *Microsoft PowerPoint* presentation.

2 Insert a new slide. Choose a slide layout with enough space for three questions and three answers on separate lines.

3 Type your questions and answers.

4 Add an animation to each answer.

5 Check your quiz slide works. Look at it as a slideshow.

My Mega Droid Quiz!

- How many legs does my robot have?
- None (he can fly!)
- Why does he have a big head?

- How does he help me after school?

 If you have time…

Use the font menu to make the answers stand out when they appear. Change their font, size or colour. Remember to make sure all the text still fits on the slide.

You will learn:

→ how to use transitions to make your presentation more interesting

→ how to use themes to make your slides more colourful.

There are lots of different effects that can make your presentation more interesting to look at.

You can choose how each slide changes to the next one. These changes are called **transitions**. If your computer has sound you can also choose a sound to go with the transition.

This will make your presentation fun and exciting.

You can also make your slides more colourful by adding themes to them.

How to add transitions to your slideshow

1 Choose the slide for your transition in the 'Slides' column.

2 Choose a transition from the menu. You can choose a different one for each slide.

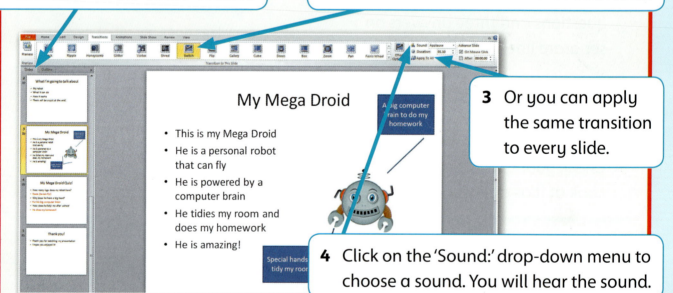

3 Or you can apply the same transition to every slide.

4 Click on the 'Sound:' drop-down menu to choose a sound. You will hear the sound.

When you have chosen all your transitions check how your presentation looks. Choose the 'From Beginning' button on the 'Slide Show' tab.

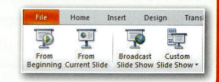

How to use a theme to make your slides more colourful

You can choose a theme for your slides. This will change the colours and fonts. Themes also add patterns and borders to your slides.

1 Select the 'Design' menu.

2 Click on a theme.

3 Use the 'Slides' column to see how each slide looks with its new theme.

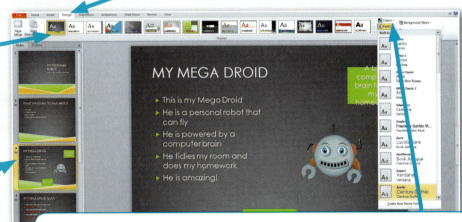

4 You can change the colours and fonts in the theme. Use the drop-down menus to make your choice.

Activity — Try out transitions and themes

1 Open your robot presentation.

2 One by one, select each slide in the 'Slides' column and add a transition.

3 Try different transitions and choose your favourite ones.

4 Choose a theme and apply it to your presentation.

5 Try different themes and choose your favourite one.

If you have time...

Customise your theme by changing the colours and fonts. Choose your favourite combination.

Talk about...

Which transitions and themes do you like best?

How do they make your presentation better?

You will learn:

→ how to print handouts for your classmates

→ how to use your slideshow to give a presentation to your class.

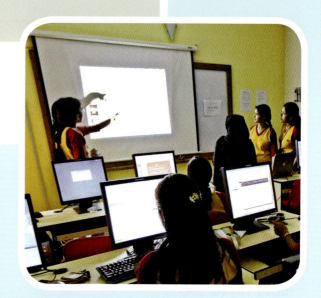

When it is time to deliver your robot presentation your slideshow must be ready on the computer you will be using.

Here are some things to remember when you deliver your presentation.

→ Know what you are going to say. You can write it down on a piece of paper.

→ Stand to the side of the screen so that everyone can see.

→ Talk slowly and clearly so that everyone in the room can hear you.

→ Change the slides as you go along. You click the left mouse button to change slides.

Handouts can help your audience understand and remember your presentation. They can show your slides or something else. Your audience can take them home with them.

How to deliver your presentation

Start your presentation with the 'From Beginning' button on the 'Slide Show' tab.

Remember that you need to click the mouse button to show the animations on your slides.

1 Use the left mouse button to change to the next slide.

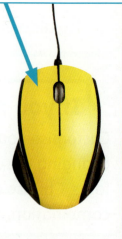

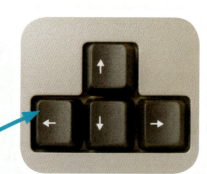

2 If you go too fast use the left arrow key on the keyboard to go back one slide.

How to print handouts for your audience

If you want to print handouts for your audience, choose 'Print' from the 'File' menu.

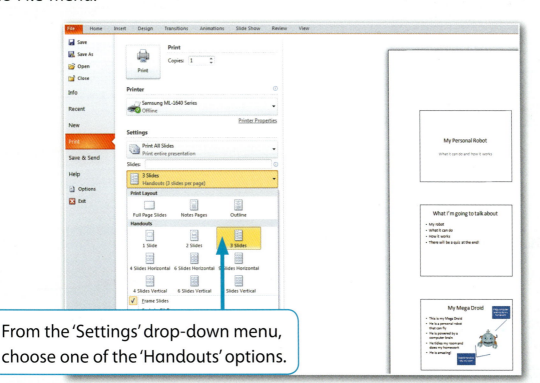

From the 'Settings' drop-down menu, choose one of the 'Handouts' options.

Activity   Deliver your presentation

1   Open your *Microsoft PowerPoint* presentation on the computer you will be using.

2   Deliver your presentation to your classmates. Talk slowly and calmly. Remember to switch to your next slide in the right place. Good luck.

 If you have time…

If your computer is connected to a printer, print handouts of your presentation for your classmates.

Talk about…

What were the best parts of your classmates' presentations? What did you enjoy about their slides?

What you have learned about multimedia

You have learned how to plan and make a slideshow to help you present your robot; make slides with words and pictures; use animations in your slideshow to make a quiz; and deliver your presentation to your classmates.

The activities on this page will let you see how much you have learned.

1 What do these words mean?

- slide

_____

- animation

_____

- transition

_____

2 Tick all of the statements that are true.

When I'm planning a presentation I should:

a include a title and an introduction ☐

b type everything I'm going to say to the audience on my slides ☐

c use text and images together ☐

d use as many animations as I can to make my slides exciting ☐

e put everything on as few slides as possible. ☐

Activity Draw a presentation

Draw a picture of a room where a presentation is happening. Include these things in your drawing and label them.

→ A presenter

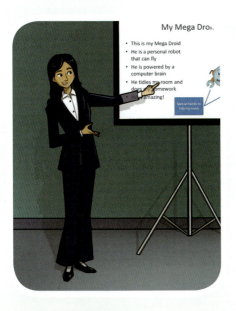

→ A screen with a slideshow

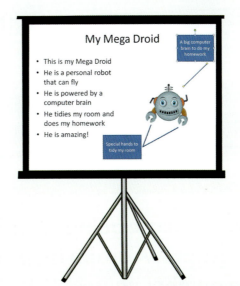

→ An audience

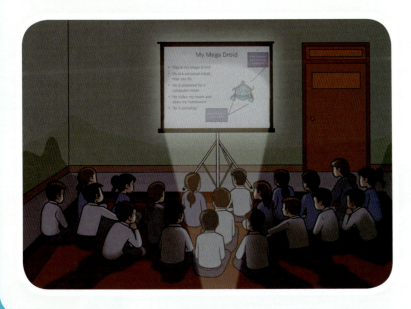

→ Some handouts

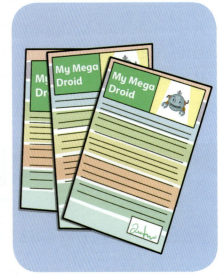

35

3 Handling data: Making graphs

By the end of this unit you will:

→ put values and labels into a spreadsheet

→ draw graphs and bar charts that show the values in the spreadsheet

→ do calculations using spreadsheet formulas

→ sort data into order.

In this unit you are going to use a spreadsheet to make graphs. A graph helps us to show and compare number values.

A spreadsheet is a type of computer software. You can enter **values** and labels. The spreadsheet can work out the answers to sums. The spreadsheet can also draw graphs for you. In this unit you will do all of these things.

Fascinating fact

Scientists study plants and develop new crops. Better crops will help to feed the people of the world.

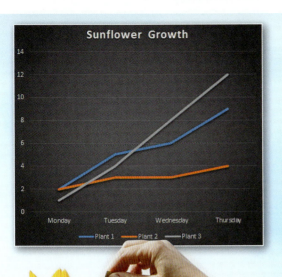

Sunflower Growth

Monday   Tuesday   Wednesday   Thursday

Plant 1   Plant 2   Plant 3

formula   key
cell reference   sort
value   bar chart
x-axis   line graph
y-axis

Talk about…

Make a class collection of graphs from magazines or the internet.

1 What information is shown in the graphs?

2 What features make graphs easy to understand?

3 Which graphs do you like best?

Activity   Collect some data

In this unit you will work with data. You can collect the data yourself.

For task one: grow three sunflowers from seed and measure their height every day.

For task two: measure the height of every student in your class.

You will learn:

→ how to make a spreadsheet by entering text and numbers.

A spreadsheet is a grid of columns and rows. The rows are numbered. The columns have letters.

Where a column crosses a row it makes a cell. The name of a cell is made of the column letter and the row number. This is called the **cell reference**.

This cell is where column C crosses row 5.

The cell reference is C5.

We use spreadsheets to store information:

→ number values

→ labels which tell us what the number values mean.

You will make a spreadsheet which records the growth of a plant.

How to put data into a spreadsheet

Select a cell by clicking on it.

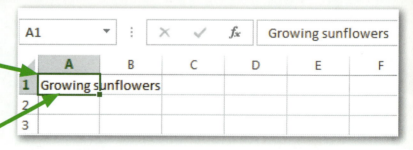

1 Cell A1 is selected.

2 Type this title and press the 'Enter' key.

Labels show the days when the plant was measured. Enter these labels into the spreadsheet.

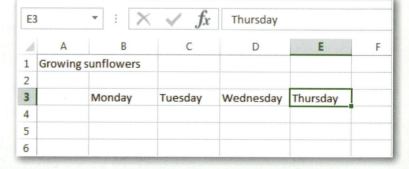

Number values show the height of the plant in centimetres. Enter these values into the spreadsheet.

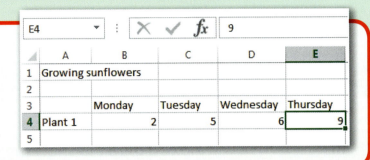

Activity Create a spreadsheet

Create a spreadsheet which looks like the example shown on this page.

You can use the data on this page to make your spreadsheet.

If you have measured a plant yourself, you can use your own data instead.

How to format text

In Unit 1 'Robots!' you learned how to format text. You learned to change the size and font. You learned how to make text bold.

You can do all these types of formatting in a spreadsheet too.

2 Use the Font menu to make the text in the cell look different.

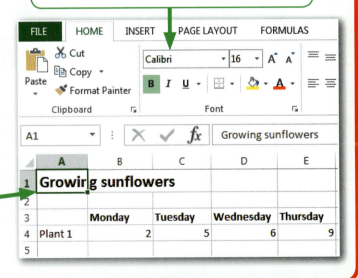

1 Select a cell.

 If you have time…

Format some of the text in your spreadsheet.

Choose the font colours, sizes and styles that you like best.

Create a line graph

You will learn:

→ how to create a graph that shows the values in a spreadsheet

→ how to choose the type and style of graph.

In this lesson you will make a graph to show the growth of the plant. You will make a **line graph**. A line graph shows the change in a value. Where the line is high the value is high. Where the line is low the value is low.

A line graph is a good way to show how much something changes over time.

How to make a graph from a spreadsheet

Select the cells you need by dragging the mouse cursor over them.

1 Click here to open the 'INSERT' tab.

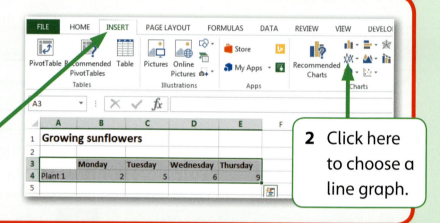

2 Click here to choose a line graph.

How to choose the style of graph

You can choose what the line graph will look like.

1 Click on the line style you want.

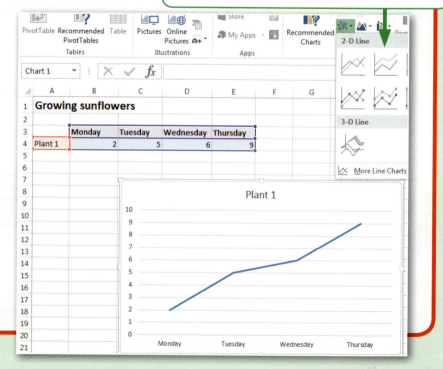

2 The graph appears on the screen.

Activity   Make a line graph

Follow the instructions on page 40 to make a line graph.

The features of a line graph

We use a line graph to show change over time. It has some important features.

The title tells us what the graph is about. This graph is about the growth of Plant 1.

The **y-axis**. This shows the measurements. In this graph it shows the height of the plant in centimetres.

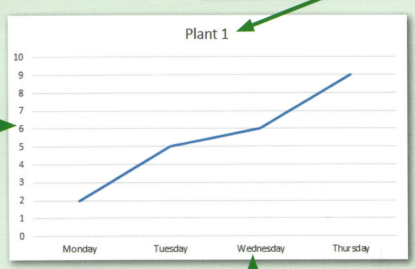

The **x-axis**. The labels on the x-axis tell us when each measurement was made. In this graph we used days.

If you have time...

Make a new graph. Select the same cells for your graph as before. Choose a different type of graph. Here is an example.

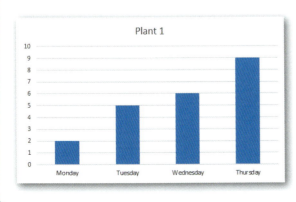

Talk about...

Look at some different types of graph. Which ones do you like best? Which graphs are easiest to understand?

You will learn:

➜ how to create a line graph with more than one line.

You have made a spreadsheet which shows the growth of one plant.

Now you will add extra labels and values.
The spreadsheet will show the growth of three plants.

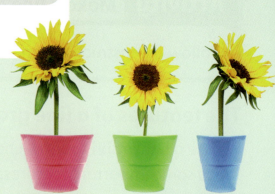

	A	B	C	D	E	F
1	**Growing sunflowers**					
2						
3		**Monday**	**Tuesday**	**Wednesday**	**Thursday**	
4	Plant 1	2	5	6	9	
5	Plant 2	2	3	3	4	
6	Plant 3	1	4	8	12	

How to make a graph with three lines

Enter the labels and values shown here.

1 Select the data by dragging the mouse cursor over the cells.

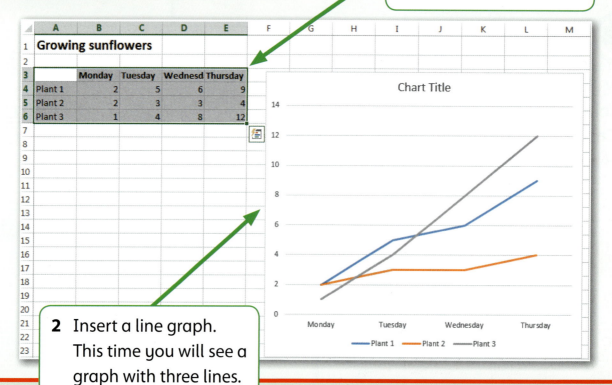

2 Insert a line graph. This time you will see a graph with three lines.

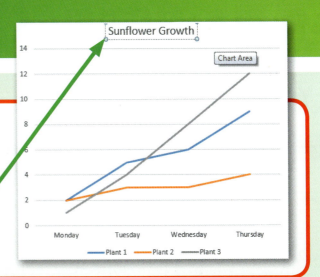

How to add a title

At the top of the graph it says 'Chart Title'.

Click on the chart title.

Type a new title.

Activity **Create a graph with three lines**

Follow the instructions on page 42 to make a line graph with three lines.

Give your graph a chart title.

 If you have time…

Experiment with different types and styles of graph. You can change the colour and other features.

Talk about…

What are the advantages of making a graph with a computer instead of drawing it yourself?

Are there any disadvantages?

The features of a graph with many lines

A line graph with more than one line has extra features.

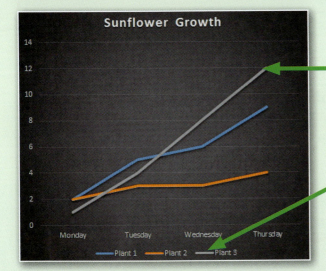

The lines are different colours so you can tell them apart.

This is called the **key** or **legend**. It tells you what the three colours mean.

You will learn:

→ how to use a formula to calculate new values
→ how to build up a formula
→ how to copy a formula.

A formula to calculate growth

We use a spreadsheet **formula** to do calculations. In this lesson you will create a spreadsheet formula. It will calculate how much Plant 1 has grown between Monday and Thursday.

We need to:

→ **start with** the height of Plant 1 on Thursday

→ **take away** the height of Plant 1 on Monday.

Remember that every cell has a name. The name of a cell is the **cell reference**.

You can put a cell reference into a formula by clicking on that cell.

We will start with a new column to put our formula.

1 Add the heading here.

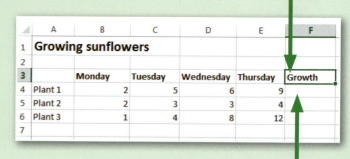

	A	B	C	D	E	F
1	Growing sunflowers					
2						
3		Monday	Tuesday	Wednesday	Thursday	Growth
4	Plant 1	2	5	6	9	
5	Plant 2	2	3	3	4	
6	Plant 3	1	4	8	12	
7						

2 The formula will go here.

How to start a formula

Every formula begins with the equals sign.

Select the cell where the formula will go. Type an equals sign.

| ▼ | : | ✕ ✓ *fx* | = |

	A	B	C	D	E	F
1	Growing sunflowers					
2						
3		Monday	Tuesday	Wednesday	Thursday	Growth
4	Plant 1	2	5	6	9	=
5	Plant 2	2	3	3	4	
6	Plant 3	1	4	8	12	
7						

How to build the formula

Here are the steps.

→ Click on the cell that shows the height on Thursday.

→ Type the take away sign.

→ Click on the cell that shows the height on Monday.

B4	▼	:	✗ ✓ fx	=E4-B4		
◢	A	B	C	D	E	F
1	Growing sunflowers					
2						
3		Monday	Tuesday	Wednesday	Thursday	Growth
4	Plant 1	2	5	6	9	=E4-B4
5	Plant 2	2	3	3	4	
6	Plant 3	1	4	8	12	
7						

When you have finished the formula press 'Enter'.

Activity Make a formula

Add a formula to your spreadsheet to calculate how much Plant 1 has grown between Monday and Thursday.

How to copy the formula

You can copy your formula down to the cells below. It will work out the values for Plant 2 and Plant 3.

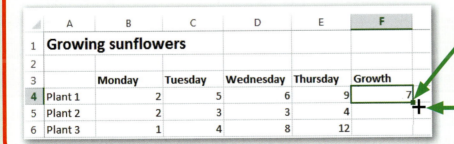

◢	A	B	C	D	E	F
1	Growing sunflowers					
2						
3		Monday	Tuesday	Wednesday	Thursday	Growth
4	Plant 1	2	5	6	9	7
5	Plant 2	2	3	3	4	
6	Plant 3	1	4	8	12	

1 Move the cursor to the corner of the cell so it looks like a cross.

2 Drag the cursor down over the other cells.

Here are the calculated values.

◢	A	B	C	D	E	F
1	Growing sunflowers					
2						
3		Monday	Tuesday	Wednesday	Thursday	Growth
4	Plant 1	2	5	6	9	7
5	Plant 2	2	3	3	4	2
6	Plant 3	1	4	8	12	11

If you have time...

Copy the formula you made down to the cells below so that it calculates the growth for Plants 2 and 3.

Create a bar chart

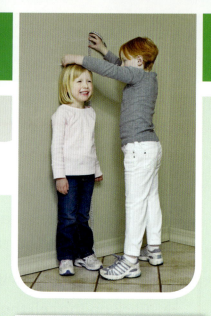

You will learn:

→ how to make a bar chart.

A **bar chart** is a graph which uses oblong bars to compare values. A bar chart is used to compare values between different people or things. In this lesson you will make a bar chart.

Preparing the data

A girl measured the height of every student in her class. She entered the names of the students into a spreadsheet. There was one name in each cell. Then she entered the students' heights into the spreadsheet.

Here is the spreadsheet that she made. You can copy this data to make your spreadsheet. Or you can use the names and heights of students in your class.

	A	B
1	**Heights in my class**	
2		
3	**Name**	**How tall (cm)**
4	Abdul	128
5	Khalid	132
6	Christopher	129
7	Rahim	118
8	Jenny	115
9	Aysha	124
10	Layla	124
11	Nathalie	122
12	Zara	123
13	Matthew	129

How to make a bar chart

You must select the data which will make the graph. Then select the graph type.

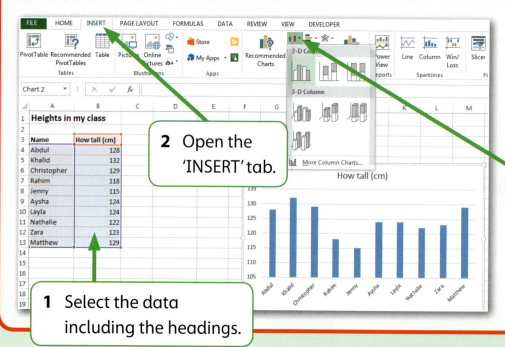

2 Open the 'INSERT' tab.

3 Select the 'bar chart' type.

1 Select the data including the headings.

Activity   Make a bar chart of heights

1   Start a new spreadsheet.

2   Enter the student names and heights shown here. Or enter data you have collected in your class.

3   Follow the instructions on this page to make a bar chart.

4   You can change the chart title if you want. (Look back at page 43.)

 If you have time…

You can change the design for your bar chart.
Click on the chart to select it.

1   Click here to open the 'DESIGN' tab.

3   You can also change the colour scheme.

2   Pick the chart style you like best.

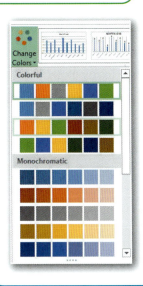

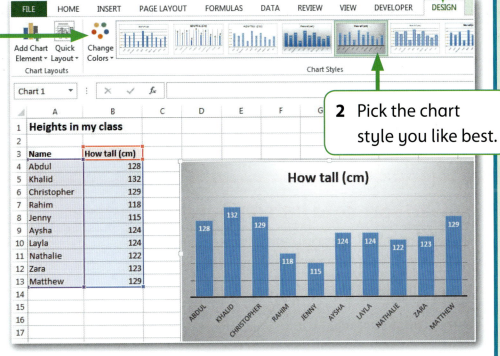

	A	B
1	**Heights in my class**	
2		
3	**Name**	**How tall (cm)**
4	Abdul	128
5	Khalid	132
6	Christopher	129
7	Rahim	118
8	Jenny	115
9	Aysha	124
10	Layla	124
11	Nathalie	122
12	Zara	123
13	Matthew	129

You will learn:

→ how to sort a table of data into alphabetical order

→ how to sort a table of data into numerical order.

> When you sort the data, the bar chart will change too. In this picture the data is sorted into name order.

You have made a spreadsheet which stores the names of students and their heights. You have made a bar chart which displays this data.

Heights in my class

Name	How tall (cm)
Abdul	128
Aysha	124
Christopher	129
Jenny	115
Khalid	132
Layla	124
Matthew	129
Nathalie	122
Rahim	118
Zara	123

In this lesson you will sort the data into

→ name order

→ height order.

Sort means to put a table of data into alphabetical order (A, B, C, …) or numerical order (1, 2, 3, …). We use one of the columns in the table to decide on the sort order.

Sorting data into order has many advantages.

→ It makes the data easier to read.

→ It is easier to find the information you want.

	A	B
1	**Heights in my class**	
2		
3	Name	How tall (cm)
4	Abdul	128
5	Khalid	132
6	Christopher	129
7	Rahim	118
8	Jenny	115
9	Aysha	124
10	Layla	124
11	Nathalie	122
12	Zara	123
13	Matthew	129

How to sort data into alphabetical order

Select the data that you want to sort. You can include the headings such as 'Name' and 'How tall (cm)'. The computer will ignore them.

The easiest sort uses the first column of a list.

1 Click on the 'Sort & Filter' button at the right of the toolbar.

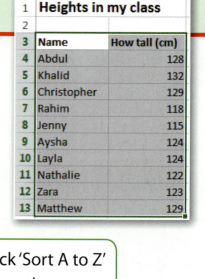

2 Pick 'Sort A to Z' from the menu.

Activity Sort your data

1 Sort the data into name order.

2 Print out the data and the bar chart.

How to sort data into numerical order

Now you will sort data into numerical order of heights.

1 Click on the 'Sort & Filter' button.

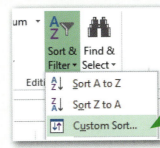

2 Pick 'Custom Sort'.

You will see a window like this.

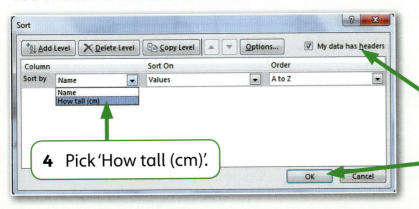

3 Make sure this box is ticked.

4 Pick 'How tall (cm)'.

5 Click on 'OK'.

If you have time...

1 Sort the data into height order.

2 Choose a design for the bar chart.

3 Print out the data and the bar chart.

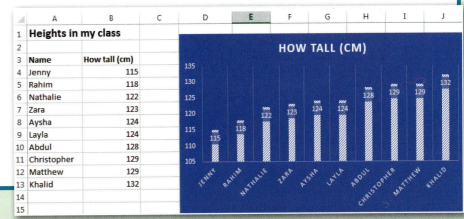

What you have learned about handling data

You have learned how to put values and labels into a spreadsheet; draw graphs and bar charts that show the values in the spreadsheets; do calculations using spreadsheet formulas; and sort data into order.

The activities on this page will let you see how much you have learned.

1   Name one advantage of showing data as a graph instead of a list of numbers.

_____

_____

2   Name two different types of graph.

_____

_____

3   Which type of graph is the best to show the following data?

   a   Showing how much a child grows between the ages of 1 and 7.

   _____

   b   Showing the number of students in a class who like different flavours of ice cream.

   _____

4   What is the purpose of a key on a graph?

_____

_____

5   What are the two ways you can sort a spreadsheet list?

_____

Activity World of Lizards graph

World of Lizards is a pet store that specialises in pet lizards. It has three different types of lizard:

1 leopard gecko

2 green anole

3 blue-tongued skink.

Here is a spreadsheet which shows how many lizards there were in the shop each year. Use the skills you have learned to make this spreadsheet.

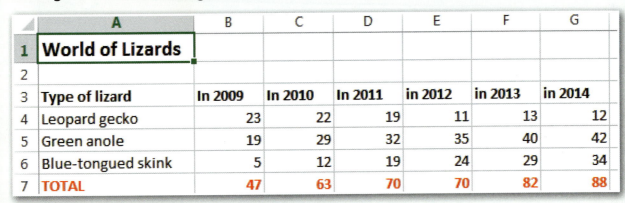

	A	B	C	D	E	F	G
1	**World of Lizards**						
2							
3	**Type of lizard**	In 2009	In 2010	In 2011	in 2012	in 2013	in 2014
4	Leopard gecko	23	22	19	11	13	12
5	Green anole	19	29	32	35	40	42
6	Blue-tongued skink	5	12	19	24	29	34
7	**TOTAL**	**47**	**63**	**70**	**70**	**82**	**88**

Now create a graph from this data.

Activity Label the graph

If you have completed the World of Lizards activity, print out your graph. If you have not completed the activity, your teacher will give you a picture of a graph.

Write on the graph to show:

1 the *x*-axis   **2** the *y*-axis   **3** the title   **4** the key

5 the line that shows how many green anoles there were in the shop.

51

4 Control the computer: The drawing bug

By the end of this unit you will:

→ know what *Scratch* is

→ know how to use *Scratch* to control the computer

→ understand the different commands that make up a *Scratch* program

→ understand how to use loops to make your programs more powerful

→ know how to get input from the user.

In this unit you will make a little bug that draws on the screen using *Scratch*.

A computer program is a set of instructions.

Computer programs control the way that a computer works. Different programs make the computer do different things.

In this unit you will use *Scratch* to create simple computer programs. Your programs will control a small image called a sprite. Your program will make the sprite move about on the screen.

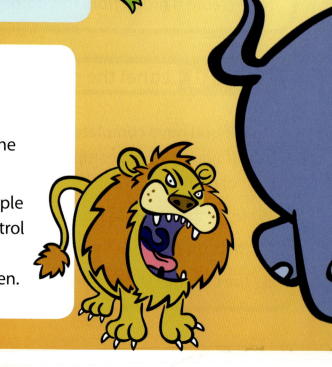

Talk about...

Discuss the computer games you have played. What objects can you control when you play these games?

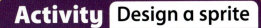

Activity Design a sprite

1 Look at the *Scratch* sprites on these pages. You will pick one of these later. You can also use images that you have made yourself!

2 On paper, draw a design for a sprite. You can make it as colourful as you like.

Computer games are programs that let you control objects on the screen. The objects can be anything: people or pieces in a game, or something else.

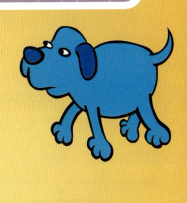

fixed loop

blocks

sprite

right-click

loop

script

Scratch

output

stage

user input

user

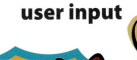

Fascinating fact

The first computers were huge! One computer could fill a large room, with hardly any space for people to fit in too!

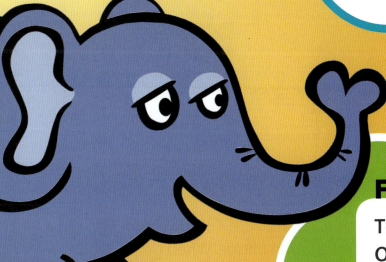

53

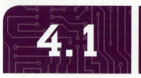

You will learn:

➜ what *Scratch* is
➜ what a sprite is
➜ how to choose a sprite.

Scratch is a programming language. When you start up *Scratch* you will see a screen like this.

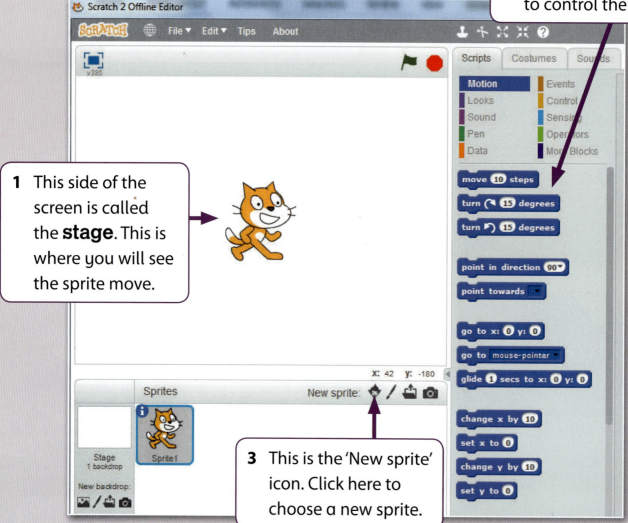

1 This side of the screen is called the **stage**. This is where you will see the sprite move.

2 This side of the screen is called the **script**. This is where you will create the program to control the sprite.

3 This is the 'New sprite' icon. Click here to choose a new sprite.

The computer program you make will control a sprite image. When you start up *Scratch* the sprite is a cat.

In the pictures in this unit you will see a sprite called 'Ladybug 1'. But you can pick any sprite you like.

How to choose a new sprite

When you click on the 'New sprite' icon you will see the Sprite Library.

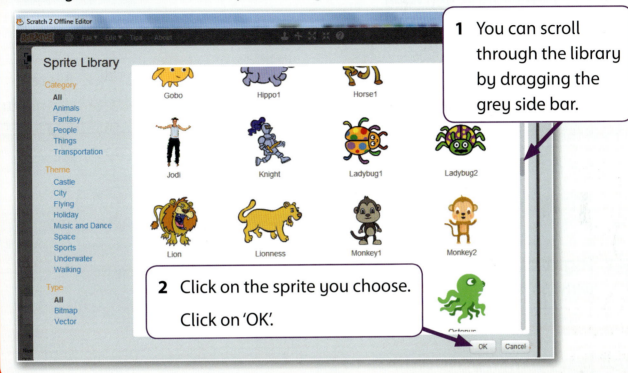

1   You can scroll through the library by dragging the grey side bar.

2   Click on the sprite you choose.

Click on 'OK'.

Activity | Choosing a sprite

1   Choose a sprite. You can pick any image you like.

2   Save your work with a suitable file name.

The program that you will make in this unit is called 'star bug'. There is a ready-made example of this program for you to look at.

If you have time...

The program that you will make in this unit is called 'star bug'. Investigate the 'star bug' program.

1   Get into pairs.

2   Look at the 'star bug' script together. See what happens when you run the program.

3   Click on the green flag to run the program.

4   Click on the red dot to stop the program.

You will learn:

➔ how to make a script from blocks
➔ how to pick the blocks you need
➔ how to fit the blocks together.

How to delete a sprite

Open the file you saved last time.

You can delete the cat sprite. You do not need it for the script to work.

1 **Right-click** on the cat sprite with the right button of the mouse.

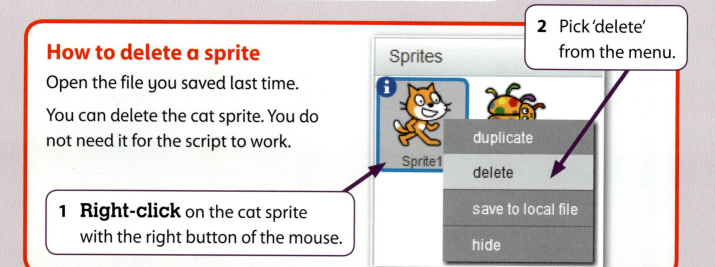

2 Pick 'delete' from the menu.

What is a *Scratch* script made of?

On pages 54–55 you picked a new sprite. Now you will make a script to control the sprite.

A *Scratch* script is made of **blocks**. They are stored in groups.

A *Scratch* script always starts with an event. So you will start with the 'event' blocks.

This star bug script will run when you click the green flag. So that is the first block to choose.

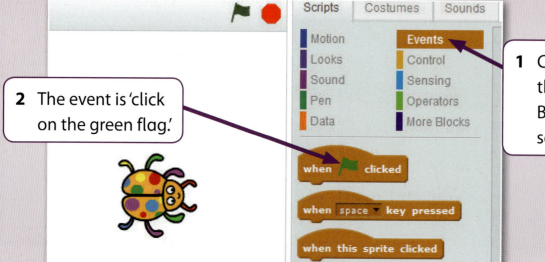

1 Click here to see the 'event' blocks. Blocks in this section are brown.

2 The event is 'click on the green flag.'

How to add a block to the script

To add a block to the script you must drag it into the script area. The blocks will join together. You can add blocks to make the sprite move forward and turn.

Motion blocks are blue. Some make the sprite walk forward. Some make the sprite turn.

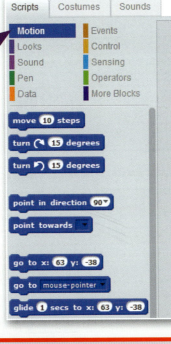

1 Click here to see the 'motion' blocks.

2 Drag the block for 'move 10 steps' onto the script area. Join it to the 'event' block.

3 Drag the block for 'turn 15 degrees' onto the script area. Join it to the other blocks.

Activity | Make a script by joining blocks together

1 Add lots of blocks, like in the picture.

2 Run the script by clicking on the green flag. Click lots of times.

3 Save your work.

 If you have time...

Experiment by adding other motion blocks to the script. See the effect of these changes.

You will learn:

→ what a loop is and why they make scripts more powerful

→ how to add a loop to your script

→ how to make the sprite draw on the screen.

On pages 56–57 you made a long script with lots of blocks in it. The same blocks were repeated over and over again.

Now you will replace that long list of blocks with a single 'loop'. A **loop** is a control that makes the script repeat.

Scripts	Costumes	Sounds

Motion — Events
Looks — Control
Sound — Sensing
Pen — Operators
Data — More Blocks

wait 1 secs

repeat 10

forever

1 The loop blocks are in the 'Control' section.

2 This loop will repeat ten times.

3 This loop will repeat forever.

How to add a loop to a script you made

Step 1

First you will delete the repeated blocks.

Pull the first blue block away from the event block. All the other blocks will come with it.

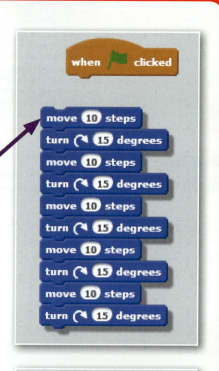

when 🚩 clicked

move 10 steps
turn ↻ 15 degrees
move 10 steps
turn ↻ 15 degrees
move 10 steps
turn ↻ 15 degrees
move 10 steps
turn ↻ 15 degrees
move 10 steps
turn ↻ 15 degrees

Now drag the joined-together blocks off the script area, back to where they came from.

Step 2

Find the 'forever' loop in the yellow control blocks area. Join it to the event block.

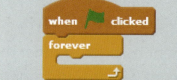

when 🚩 clicked

forever

Step 3

Open the blue 'motion' blocks. You need one 'move' block and one 'turn' block.

> Put the blocks inside the forever loop.

The forever loop will make the blocks repeat forever.

How to make the sprite draw a line with a pen

The sprite can draw a line. The green 'pen' blocks control this. Add these blocks to the script.

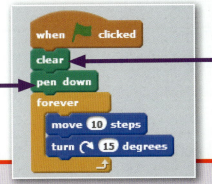

2 'Pen down' will make the sprite draw with a pen.

1 'Clear' will clear the screen when the script starts.

Activity | Create a loop in your script

1 Using the instructions on these pages, add a loop to your script.

2 Add blocks so that the sprite draws with a pen.

3 Run the script. See what shape the sprite draws.

4 To stop the script, click the red dot. Save your work.

When you run a computer program it produces a result. In this example the result was a drawing of a star. The result of a computer program is called the **output** of the program.

Talk about...

What computer outputs can you think of?

You will learn:

→ why script blocks contain values

→ how to change the values in the script blocks

→ what happens when you change script values.

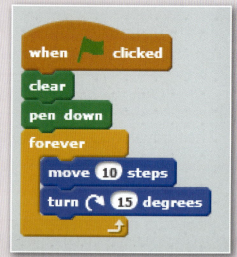

On pages 58–59 you used a loop to control the sprite.

The sprite will keep moving until you stop the program.

You also added a pen to the script. The sprite will draw a line when it moves.

Changing number values

Look at the script you made. The blue motion blocks include number values.

Now you will change the number values. This will change what the sprite does. The path it draws will change.

The first value shows how many steps the sprite walks. In *Scratch* each step is very small.

The second value sets the amount the sprite turns. It is given as a number of **degrees**.

The bigger the number of degrees, the more the sprite will turn. 90 degrees is a right angle.

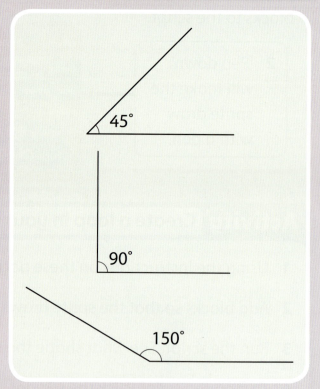

How to change number values

1 Click in the box where the number is shown.

2 Type the new number.

Activity Changing the path of the sprite using number values

1 This value sets the number of steps. Change it to 100.

2 This value sets the number of degrees. Change it to 150.

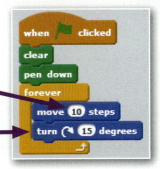

The path of the sprite should change. The new path will look like a star.

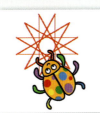

Activity Changing the colour of the pen

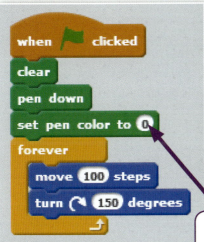

Now change the colour of the pen.

1 Select the 'pen' blocks.

2 Find the block which says 'set pen colour to 0'.

3 Drag this block into the script.

4 Make sure the script blocks show the right number values. Run the script. Save your work.

This value sets the colour of the pen. It can be any value from 0 to 300.

If you have time...

Change the number values in the script blocks. Explore the effect of entering different number values. You can make the sprite draw many different shapes in different colours.

You will learn:

➔ what a fixed loop is

➔ how to use a fixed loop in programming

➔ how to make a rainbow image.

The commands inside the loop repeat forever.

Another kind of loop is a fixed loop. A **fixed loop** will repeat a fixed number of times. Then it will stop.

A fixed loop is also called a counter-controlled loop. That is because the computer counts how many times it repeats.

How to make a fixed loop

Look at the script you made. Pull the blocks apart from each other. Drag the 'forever loop' piece back to the blocks area.

```
when [flag] clicked
clear
pen down
set pen color to 0

forever

        move 100 steps
        turn ↻ 150 degrees
```

Look in the 'Control' section. Find the block that says 'repeat 10'. Drag this block to the script area. Make the script using this block.

It will look like the picture here.

1 This block will repeat the loop ten times.

```
when [flag] clicked
clear
pen down
set pen color to 0
repeat 10
    move 150 steps
    turn ↻ 280 degrees
```

2 Change the values as shown here.

When you run the script the sprite will draw this image.

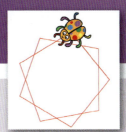

How to make a rainbow star

Look in the 'Pen' section. Find the block that says 'change pen colour by 10'. Drag it into the loop. Now every time the loop repeats the pen colour will change.

```
when      clicked
clear
pen down
set pen color to 0
repeat 100
    move 150 steps
    turn ↻ 190 degrees
    change pen color by 10
```

3 Change the number of steps to 150.

2 Change the number of repeats to 100.

4 Change the number of degrees to 190.

1 The new block goes here.

When you run the script the sprite will draw this image.

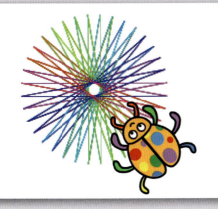

Activity Practise the scripts

1 Make the two scripts shown on this page.

2 Run the scripts to see what they do.

If you have time...

Make more changes to the scripts. Experiment with the two different types of loop.

Talk about...

In *Scratch* the different types of block are different colours.

1 What colours are used?

2 How does the use of colour help you to learn?

You will learn:

➔ what user input is
➔ why user input is useful
➔ how to add user input to a script.

The **user** is the person who controls the program. The user makes the program stop and start.

User input means the values that the user types while the program is running. In this lesson you will write a script which asks the user for input.

How to add input as a user

Step 1

Look in the 'Motion' section of the block area. Find the block that looks like this picture.

```
go to x: -59 y: 68
```

1 These numbers may be different.

Drag the block into your script at the very top. This sets the position of the sprite at the start of the program.

```
when [flag] clicked
go to x: 0 y: 0
clear
pen down
set pen color to 0
repeat 100
    move 150 steps
    turn ↻ 190 degrees
    change pen color by 10
```

2 Change the values to 0 as shown here. The sprite will start in the very middle of the screen.

Step 2

Look in the 'Sensing' section of the block area.
Find the block that looks like this picture.
This block will ask the user a question.
Change the question from 'What's your name?'
to 'How many degrees?'

`ask` `What's your name?` `and wait`

> **1** Drag the block into the script before the loop.

```
when [flag] clicked
go to x: 0 y: 0
clear
pen down
set pen color to 0
ask How many degrees? and wait
repeat 100
    move 150 steps
    turn ↻ 190 degrees
    change pen color by 10
```

When you run the program the sprite will ask you the question.

`answer`

Step 3

Look at the place where you found the question block. You will find an answer block.

This block will store the answer that the user typed in.

Drag the block into your script in the position shown here. It fits into another block.

```
when [flag] clicked
go to x: 0 y: 0
clear
pen down
set pen color to 0
ask How many degrees? and wait
repeat 100
    move 150 steps
    turn ↻ answer degrees
    change pen color by 10
```

Activity | Entering different numbers

1 Run the script you have built.

2 Try entering different numbers and see how the image changes.

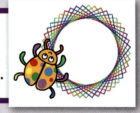

 If you have time...

See if you can change the script so that instead of asking the number of degrees it asks the number of steps.

What you have learned about controlling the computer

You have learned how to control a sprite; how to make a script out of blocks; how to use a loop to repeat commands; how to change values; and how to include user input.

The activities on this page will let you see how much you have learned.

1 What is a *Scratch* script?

_____

_____

2 What are *Scratch* blocks used for?

_____

_____

3 A *Scratch* program included the command 'pen down'. What does that command do?

_____

4 What happens to *Scratch* commands that are in a loop?

_____

5 What is the difference between a 'forever' loop and a fixed loop?

_____

6 What is user input?

_____

Activity — Label the picture

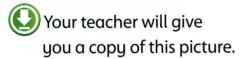

⬇ Your teacher will give you a copy of this picture.

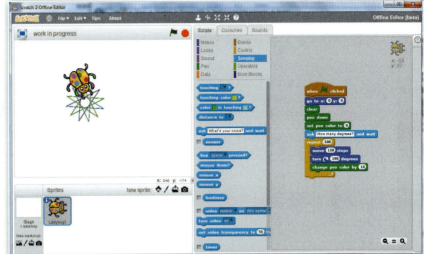

Write on the picture to show:

→ Where the script is.

→ Where the sprite is.

→ Where you click to make the program start.

→ Where you click to make the program stop.

Activity — Make a forever loop for a *Scratch* sprite

1 Pick a *Scratch* sprite.

2 Create a script for the sprite which will make it go forward 150 steps and turn 145 degrees.

3 Put these commands inside a 'forever' loop.

⏱ If you have time...

Extend the script you created in the last activity so that your sprite draws a rainbow star.

Here is one that shows a cat sprite drawing a rainbow star.

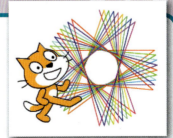

67

5 The internet: Communicating online

By the end of this unit you will:

→ send and receive an email

→ send an email attachment

→ find an email

→ keep yourself safe when you use email.

In this unit you are going to use email to write an adventure story with a partner.

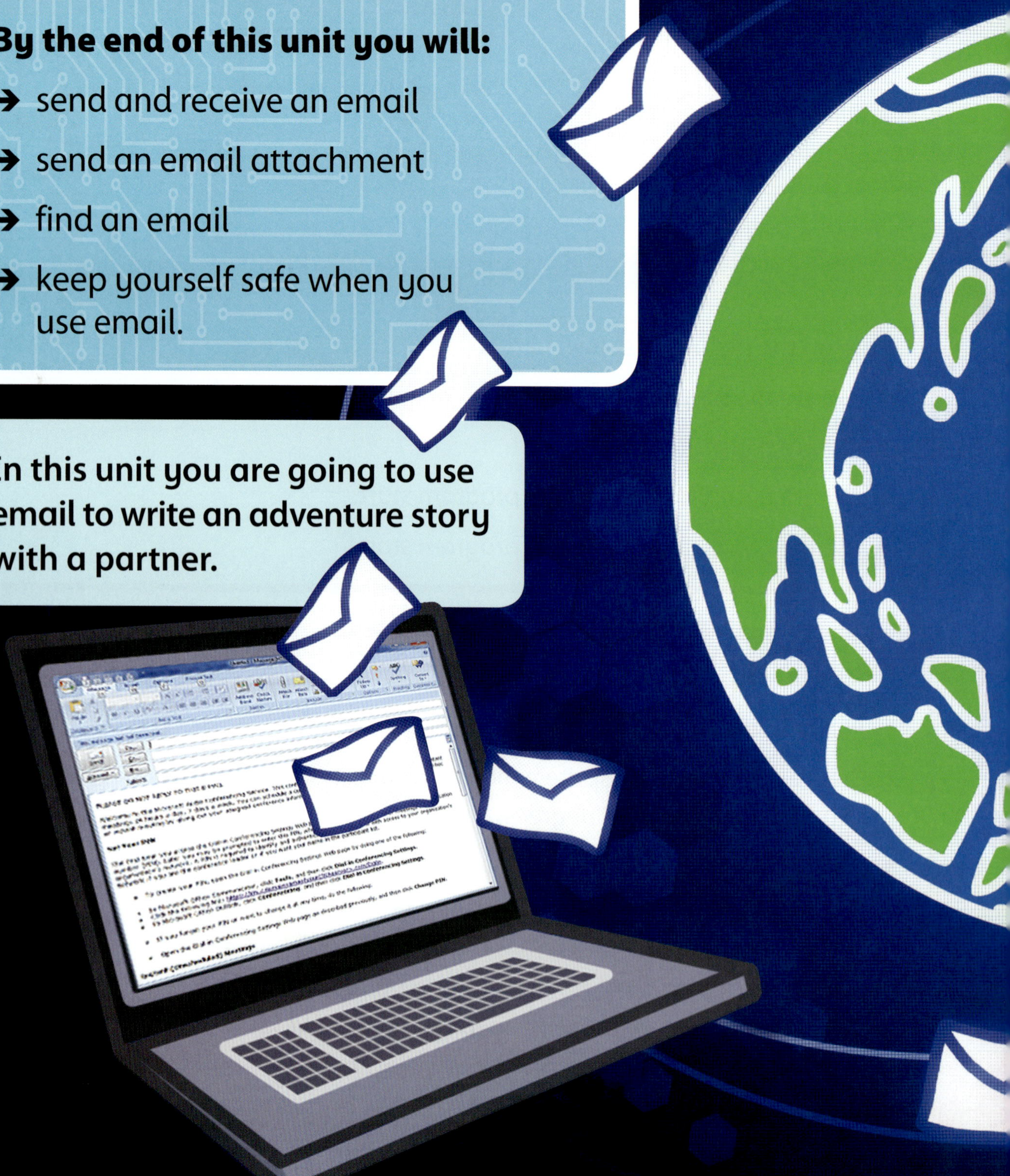

virus protection
attachment phishing
spoofing pharming
spam email

People have been writing letters for thousands of years. Papyrus letters have been found in Egypt that are 3000 years old. Even older messages on clay have been found in what was ancient Mesopotamia.

Talk about...

Why is it useful to communicate by writing as well as talking?

Fascinating fact

In ancient Mesopotamia people wrote using reeds. They pressed the reeds into wet clay. This kind of writing is called 'cuneiform'.

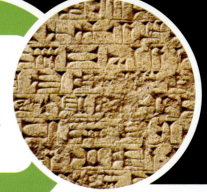

You will learn:

➔ about different ways of communicating
➔ what email is
➔ why email is popular.

Talk about...

Have you ever written or received a letter?

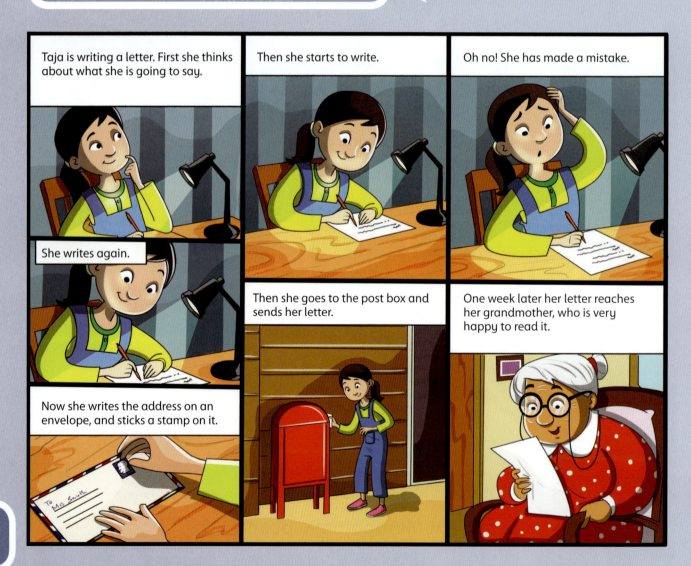

Taja is writing a letter. First she thinks about what she is going to say.

Then she starts to write.

Oh no! She has made a mistake.

She writes again.

Now she writes the address on an envelope, and sticks a stamp on it.

Then she goes to the post box and sends her letter.

One week later her letter reaches her grandmother, who is very happy to read it.

Many people love to get letters. But sometimes we need to send a message more quickly. We can use electronic mail – called **email** – to send messages in an instant.

We can communicate in lots of different ways. To communicate means to share ideas or information with another person.

→ Some ways of communicating are very reliable. Reliable means that the message will definitely get to the other person.

→ Some ways are very quick.

→ Some ways are easy to use. Some ways are very popular.

Activity Ways of communicating

Your teacher will give you a worksheet. Look at the different ways of communicating.

→ Is each way of communicating:

– reliable?   – quick?   – easy to use?

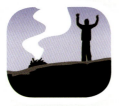 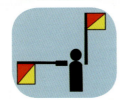 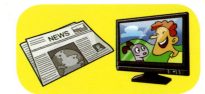 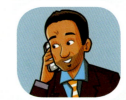

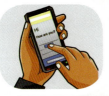 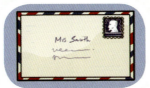 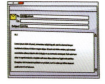 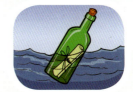

→ Do people like this way of communicating?

Draw faces to show what you think.

Talk about…

Compare your faces with a partner. Are they the same?

Why do you think email is so popular?

If you have time…

Can you make up your own way of communicating?

You will learn:

➜ about the different parts of an email.

Emails and letters are similar in some ways, and different in others.

This is a letter.

Oxford International Primary Computing | Student Book 3

LESSON 5.2 Worksheet

Hilltop Cottage
Green Knoll Town
Happy State
LT12 7834

19 April

Dear student,

I have heard you are a famous explorer.

Please can you help me find an ancient lost clay tablet. It has a wonderful story written on it in a mysterious language.

The tablet is quite heavy. You will need to find a way to bring it home safely. I know it is in a distant country. I need a brave adventurer to travel there to fetch it.

Please can you make the trip and find the tablet?

Thank you!

Yours sincerely,
Your friend

© Oxford University Press 2014

1 This is the header. It has the address and the date.

2 This is the greeting.

3 This is the body.

4 This is the closing.

5 This is the signature.

This is an email.

Oxford International Primary Computing | Student Book 3

From: me@mysteriouslanguages.com
To: student@adventure.com
Date: 19 April 09:46
Subject: Ancient clay tablet

Dear student,

I have heard you are a famous explorer.

Please can you help me find an ancient lost clay tablet. It has a wonderful story written on it in a mysterious language.

The tablet is quite heavy. You will need to find a way to bring it home safely. I know it is in a distant country. I need a brave adventurer to travel there to fetch it.

Please can you make the trip and find the tablet?

Thank you!

Kind regards,
Your friend

© Oxford University Press 2014

1 This is the email address.

2 This is the time and date the email was sent.

3 This is the subject.

4 This is the body.

5 This is the signature. An email has an electronic signature. It can include an image, a quote or information about the sender.

Activity [Email jigsaw]

 Look at the worksheet your teacher has given you.

Complete the email so that all the parts of the email are in the right places.

Oxford International Primary Computing | Student Book 3

UNIT 5.2 Worksheet
Email jigsaw

Can you stick the parts of the email into the correct places?
Write in today's date and the time now.
Write in your signature.

To:	
Subject:	
Date and time:	
Greeting:	
Body:	
Signature:	

You will need to pack lots of things for your adventure. Don't forget to pack the right clothes and shoes, equipment and food. Let me know if you need any help.

Hello!

sunnyday@home.com

Things to pack for the trip

© Oxford University Press 2014

🕐 If you have time...

What is the best way to send different messages? Talk with a friend about different kinds of messages and the best ways to send them. For example, telephone, talking face-to-face or a letter.

Talk about...

With your partner, decide where your adventure is going to take place. Where are you going to search for the clay tablet?

➔ a jungle?

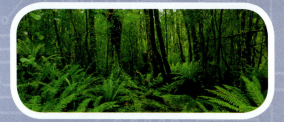

➔ a polar ice cap?

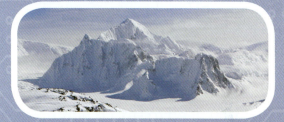

➔ a desert?

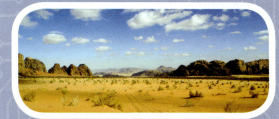

➔ an ocean?

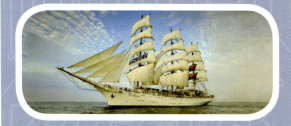

You will learn:

→ how to send and receive an email.

Email addresses

All email addresses look similar.
For example:

1 This part is your user name.

name@place.com

2 @ means 'at'

3 This part can be a place like a school or a business, or it might be the email provider.

4 This shows where the sender is from or what kind of organisation they are in.

.com means a company.

Other examples are:

.gov means a government

.org means an organisation.

How to send an email

First you need to start a new email. Different email providers do this in different ways.

Click 'Compose', 'New' or 'New Message'.

1 Type the email address you are sending to here.

2 Type the subject of the email here. You could type 'Adventure story'.

3 Type the beginning of your story here. For example: 'I put my rucksack on my back, and started walking'.

4 Click 'Send'.

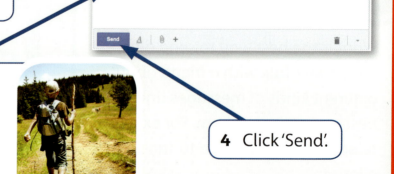

74

How to open and reply to an email

To open an email, click on the email you would like to see.

| ☐ ☆ me | **Adventure Story** - I put my rucksack on my back, and started walking. I felt nervous, but I knew I was going to do the | 11:16 am |

To reply to an email, click on the word 'Reply' or on the Reply icon.

Type your email and click 'Send'.

← REPLY

Activity Send and receive mail

Work with a partner. Take turns to type one sentence of the adventure story and then immediately email it to the other person.

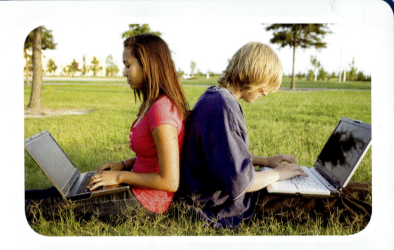

If you have time...

Can you find your sent email folder? Look at the menu on the left-hand side of your screen.

Click 'Sent Mail' or 'Sent Items'. What can you see?

Your email account usually keeps a copy of your email. You can find it in your 'Sent Items' folder.

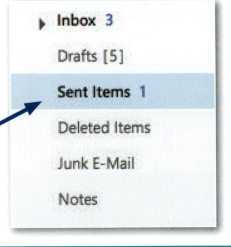

> ▸ Inbox **3**
> Drafts **[5]**
> Sent Items **1**
> Deleted Items
> Junk E-Mail
> Notes

You will learn:

→ what attachments are
→ how to send and open an attachment.

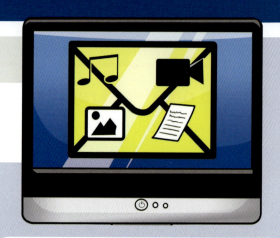

An **attachment** is an extra file that you send with an email. It can be a:

→ photograph
→ document
→ sound file
→ video.

Talk about...

Why do you think the attachment symbol is a paperclip?

How to send an email with an attachment

Click 'Compose', 'New' or 'New Message'.

1 Type the email address you are sending to here.

2 Type the subject of the email here.

3 Type the next sentence of your story here.

4 Click the paperclip symbol. It means 'attachment'.

A dialogue box will open.

Choose the file you would like to attach.

Double-click on the file, or choose 'Attach' or 'Open'.

Click 'Send'.

Activity Attach a file

Work with your partner.

Send each other an email with the next sentence of your story.
Attach a photograph to your email.

 Your teacher will show you where to find photograph files.

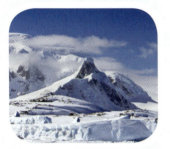
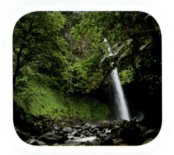
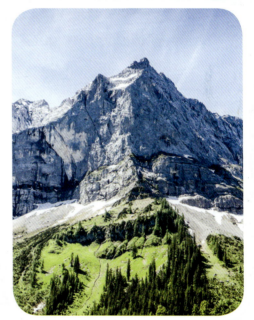
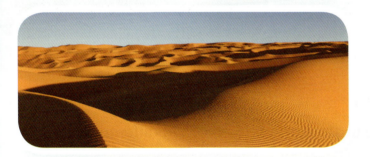
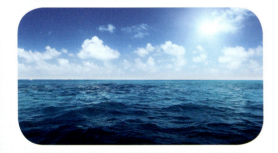
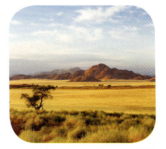
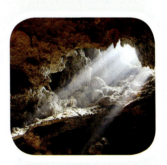

 If you have time…

Can you think of any problems with sending
some kinds of files, for example video?

You will learn:

→ how to find an email.

This is an archive. An archive is a place where people store lots of old papers.

You can create an archive for your old emails on your computer. But most email providers will store your emails for you.

You can store emails so that you can find them again another time.

Talk about...

Why is it useful to be able to find emails from the past?

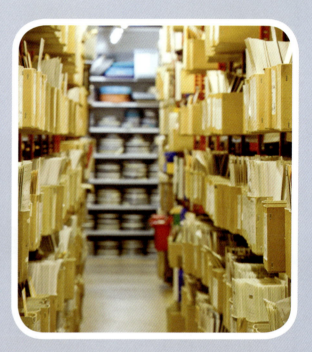

How to store and find emails

Different email providers help you to store and find emails in different ways.

To store an email, you can create folders. Some email providers call these 'labels'.

To search for an email, you can use the search box. Look for this symbol.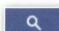

1 Type the sender's name or a key word here.

2 Then click here or press the 'Enter' key.

You can also click on your folders until you find the email you are looking for.

Activity Find an email

Can you find the email that your partner sent to you with an attachment?

Activity Continue your story

Continue your story. You will complete it in the next lesson, so make sure it is getting close to the end.

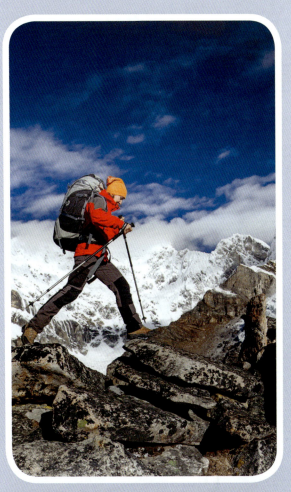

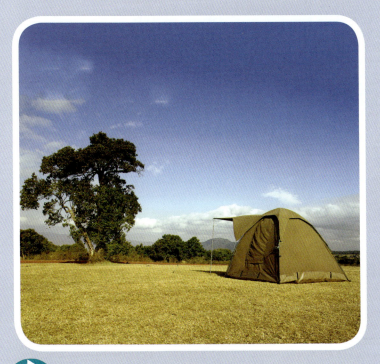

If you have time...

Can you work out how to set up a new folder in your email Inbox?

Once you have set up your folder, move all of your story emails into the folder so that you can find them easily.

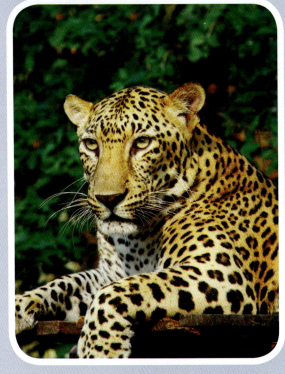

You will learn:

→ what spam, spoofing, phishing and pharming are

→ that you should never open a suspicious email

→ how to keep yourself safe when you use email.

Most people use email to communicate with other people.

Sadly, some people use email to do nasty things.

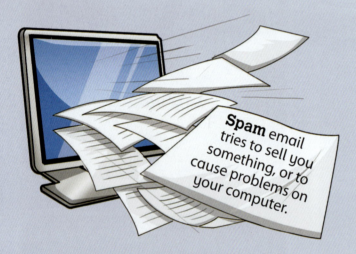

Spam email tries to sell you something, or to cause problems on your computer.

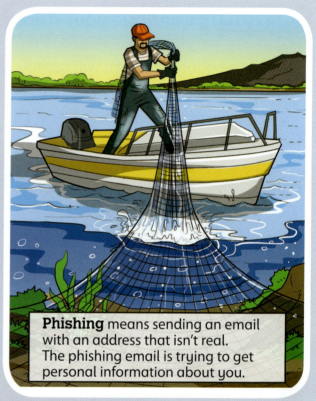

Phishing means sending an email with an address that isn't real. The phishing email is trying to get personal information about you.

Spam and phishing emails use **spoofing** to try to hide who the message really comes from.

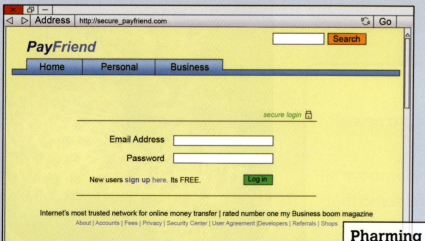

Talk about...

Why do you think people use email to do nasty things?

Pharming emails send you to a fake website.

How to keep safe from email attacks

What can we do to protect ourselves from these attacks?

Keep it closed!

Never open emails that look a bit strange, or have a strange subject. If you do not recognise the sender, do not open the email. Show it to an adult you trust.

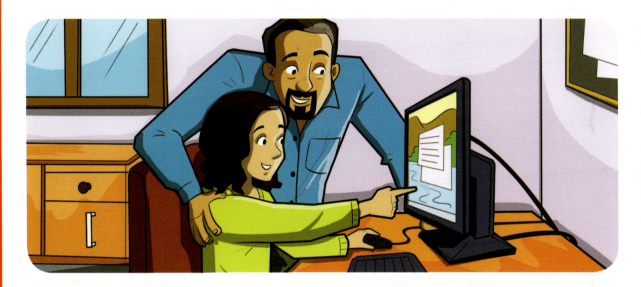

Protect!

Make sure your computer has good **virus protection**. This is software that prevents problems on your computer. It also finds problems and takes them away.

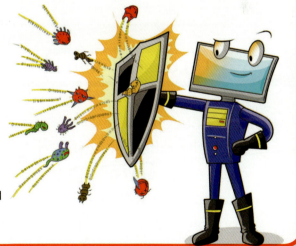

Do not reply!

Never reply to an email from someone you don't know.

Activity Finishing your story

Work with your partner to finish your email story.

 If you have time…

Make a poster about how to keep safe from email attacks.

What you have learned about the internet

You have learned about email; how to send and receive email; how to store and find your emails; and how to keep your email account and yourself safe. The activities on this page will let you see how much you have learned.

1 Write three differences between an email and a letter.

_____

_____

_____

2 What are the three ways you can keep your email account and yourself safe?

_____

_____

_____

Activity Label an email

Can you remember what the different parts of an email are called? Your teacher will give you this picture. Label the four main parts of the email.

a

c

d

b

Oxford International Primary Computing   Student Book 3

What you have learned Worksheet

From: me@mysteriouslanguages.com

To: student@adventure.com

Date: Friday July 04, 12.47 pm

Subject: Ancient story

Hello!

I have decoded the story on the clay tablet! Would you like to come to my house and hear the wonderful story we have found? I hope you will enjoy it as much as I have.

Your friend

© Oxford University Press 2014

82

Activity Send an email

Show your teacher how to send an email by putting these instructions in the correct order.

a Write the email.

b Click 'Send'.

c Write the address.

d Click 'New Message'.

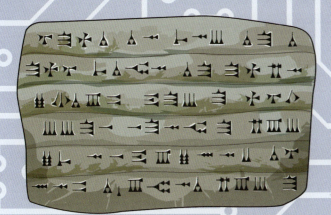

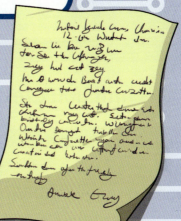

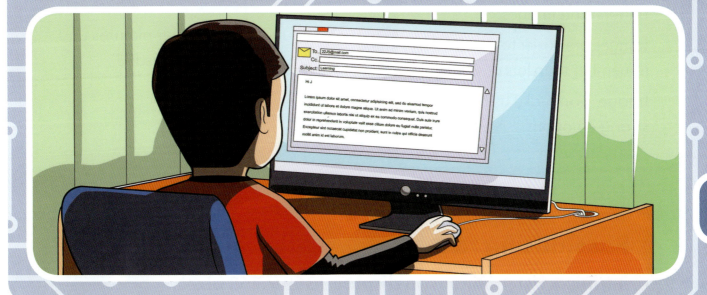

6 Computers in society: The world of pixels

By the end of this unit you will:

→ know that digital images are made of pixels

→ use pixels to measure images

→ understand that each pixel has a Red, Green, Blue value

→ learn how a computer recognises an image

→ know why digital images are important in society.

In this unit you are going to make a picture mosaic.

Pictures, also called **images**, are very powerful.

People who cannot read can understand images.

Images are easier to remember than lots of words.

Images can make us feel strong emotions.

Activity | What's in the picture?

Look at the image on this page.

1 How many colours can you see in it?

2 What are the smaller pictures you can see inside the mosaic?

Fascinating fact

A typical HD monitor can display 1366 × 768 pixels.

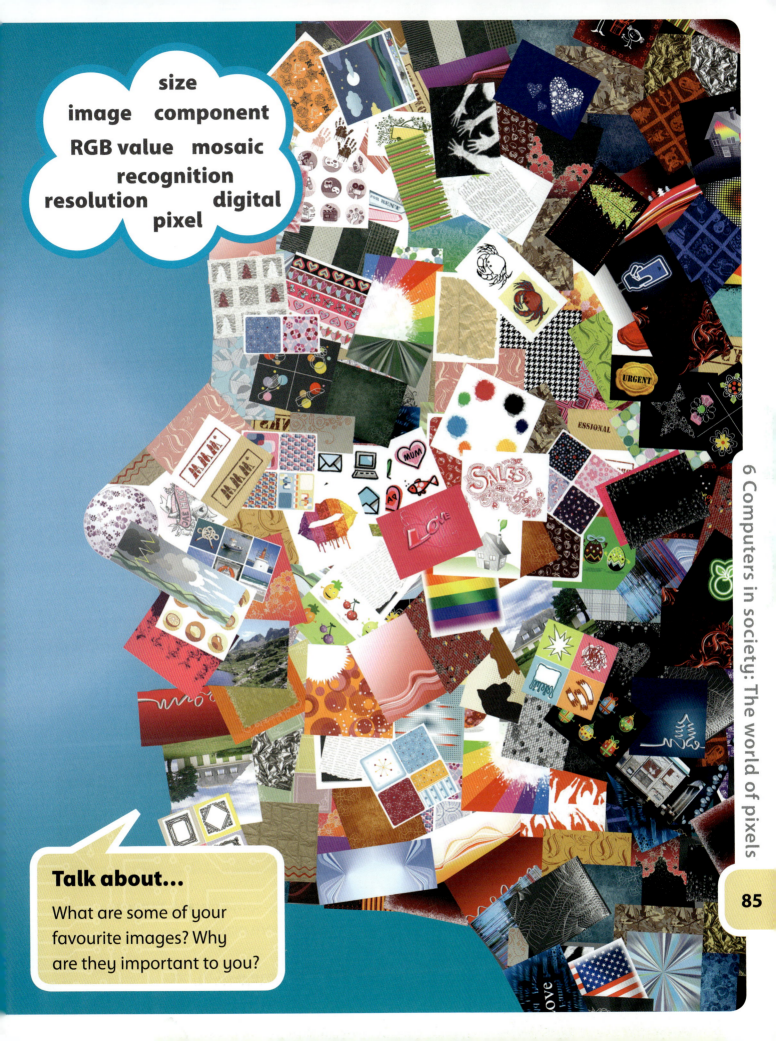

size
image   component
RGB value   mosaic
recognition
resolution   digital
pixel

Talk about...

What are some of your favourite images? Why are they important to you?

You will learn:

➔ how digital pictures are made

➔ what pixels are and how they work.

Look at this picture.

Look a little closer.

And a little closer still.

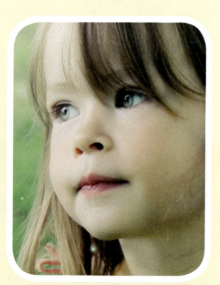 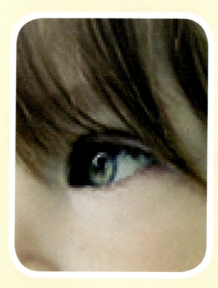 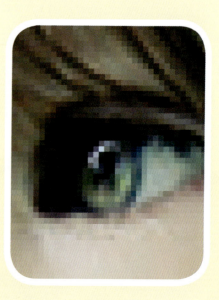

What do you see?

When we look at a **digital** picture, we actually see thousands or millions of tiny blocks of colour.

These blocks of colour are called **pixels**.

1 Digital is a word we use to talk about modern computer technology. It means the way technology deals with information.

2 'Pixel' is short for 'picture element'.

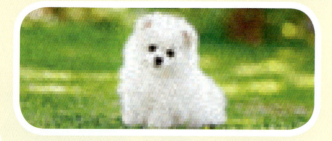 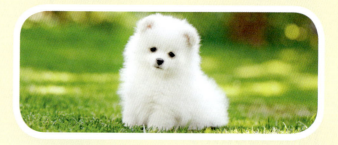

▲ What is in this picture? There are not many pixels to help us.

▲ This is the same picture, but with many more pixels.

The more pixels there are, the more the picture looks like the real thing.

Using dots to make a picture

Many years ago painters used a technique called pointillism that worked just like pixels. They used thousands of small dots to make pictures.

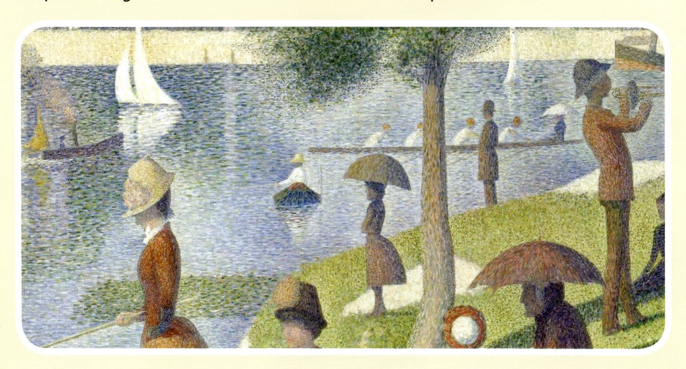

▲ Detail from *A Sunday Afternoon on the Island of La Grande Jatte*, by Georges Seurat.

Activity Going dotty

Draw something that represents your favourite activity. Use lots and lots of little dots to make your picture.

➔ If you love football, you could draw a ball.

➔ If you love reading, you could draw a book.

➔ If you love cooking, you could draw a cake.

 If you have time…

Look at the pictures your classmates are drawing. Make a list of activities that many people like.

You will learn:

➜ how we measure digital images.

Pixels are often tiny squares, but they don't have to be. They can be dots or lines.

Squares are easiest to measure.

How to measure the size of an image

We measure the **size** of an image in columns and rows of pixels.

These are columns.

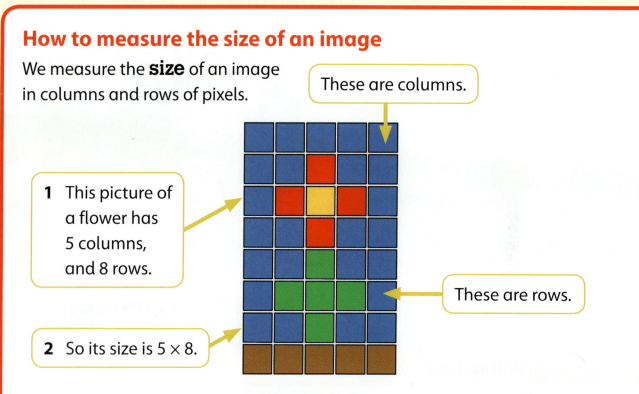

1 This picture of a flower has 5 columns, and 8 rows.

2 So its size is 5 × 8.

These are rows.

The number of pixels used to make an image is called the **resolution.**

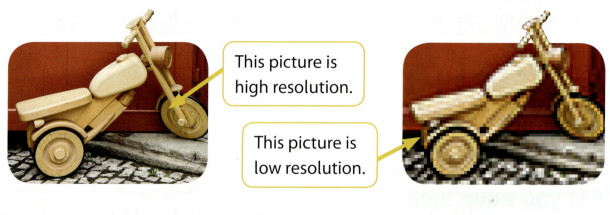

This picture is high resolution.

This picture is low resolution.

Images on computer screens or televisions have hundreds or thousands of rows and columns.

A **mosaic** is a picture made of blocks of colour or smaller pictures.

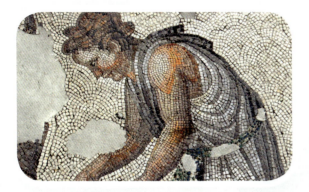

▲ This is a very old mosaic.

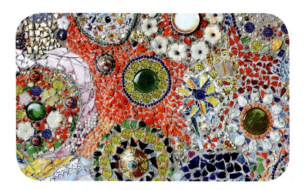

▲ This is a very new mosaic.

Activity Start your group mosaic

You are going to make a picture mosaic. Your mosaic will be about something you are interested in.

1 In your group, talk about these questions and agree what you will do.
   → Will you use squares, dots or lines for your pixels?
   → How many columns and rows will you have?
   → How big or small will your pixels be?

2 Choose one of the pictures you drew in the last lesson to make into your big mosaic.

3 Make your big sheet of paper into a grid using a ruler and a pencil.

Talk about...

Why is it easier to arrange pixels when they are squares, compared to round pixels or lines?

 If you have time...

It is easy to lay out small squares in columns and rows. Which other shapes are easy to lay out?

You will learn:

➜ what a pixel is made of

➜ that mixing RGB colours is different from mixing paint colours.

A pixel is made up of three numbers:

➜ a Red number

➜ a Green number

➜ a Blue number.

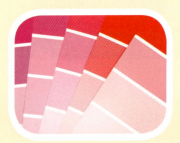

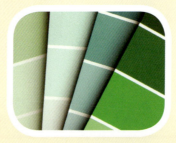

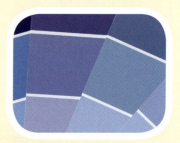

1 These are all shades of red.

2 These are all shades of green.

3 These are all shades of blue.

Normally we use a lower-case letter to write colours, but when we are writing about pixels, we use upper-case letters to write Red, Green and Blue.

When these three colours come together they make coloured pixels.

Have you ever mixed colours when you were painting?

You probably found that:

➜ Red + Blue + Yellow = Brown

➜ Red + Yellow = Orange

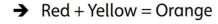

➜ Blue + Yellow = Green

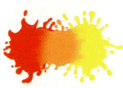

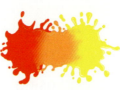

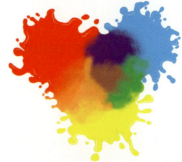

➜ Blue + Red = Purple

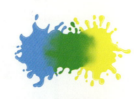

When we use RGB numbers to make colours digitally, we mix them in a different way.

Each pixel has three dots of colour from Red, Green and Blue.

The three colours are superimposed – that means they are put on top of each other. Each of the three colours is a **component** of the final colour we see with our eyes.

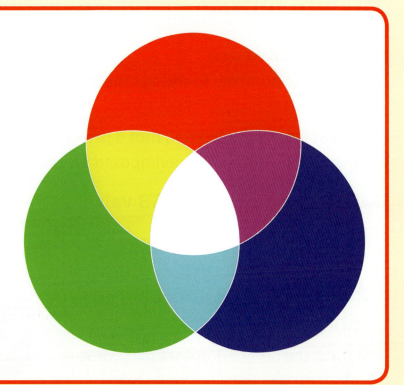

Activity   RGB colour mixing

Use the RGB colour diagram to find out which colours these mixes make.

→ Green + Blue =

→ Red + Green =

→ Red + Blue =

→ Red + Blue + Green =

Activity   Sketch your mosaic

Use the grid you drew in the last lesson to prepare your mosaic. On the grid, sketch the outlines of your picture. This will help you to create your big mosaic. It does not have to be a detailed drawing.

 If you have time…

How do you think our eyes see colour?

You will learn:

→ what an RGB value is
→ how to use numbers to change the colour of a pixel.

In the last lesson you learned that a pixel is made up of a Red, Green and Blue number, superimposed on each other.

The numbers are called the **RGB value**.

Talk about...

If Red is set to 0, it means there is no red in the pixel.

If all of the numbers are set to 0, what colour do you think you will see?

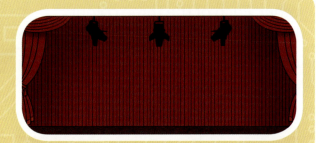

If Red is set to 255, it means there is as much red as there can be in the pixel.

If all of the numbers are set to 255, what colour do you think you will see?

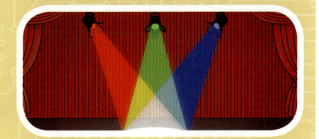

Look at this chart. Each block of colour has three numbers on it. The top number is the Red value, the middle number is the Green value, the bottom number is the Blue value.

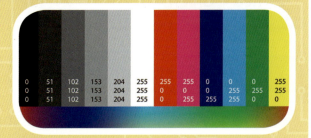

Usually, we write the RGB numbers in a row. For example:

| **1** This number is Red. | → **255, 0, 0** ← | **3** This number is Blue. |

2 This number is Green.

So the colour is Red.

Activity | Rainbow colours

The colours of the rainbow are:

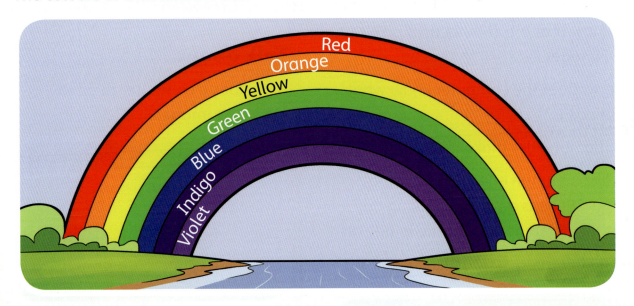

Work in your group to fit these numbers to the correct colours in the rainbow.

255, 0, 0	143, 0, 255	0, 0, 255	255, 127, 0

0, 255, 0	255, 255, 0	75, 0, 130

Activity | Make your 'pixels'

Work in your group. Start cutting or tearing coloured paper to make your picture mosaic. Which shades of colours are you going to use?

 If you have time...

Can you work out why the rainbow colours have these RGB values?

Use the Venn diagram on page 91 to help you.

You will learn:

→ how computers recognise images.

You know that a computer uses pixels to show images.

But how does the computer know what the image is?

Even human eyes make mistakes.

Just like a human eye and brain, the computer needs a way of working out what the different parts of the image are.

We call this image **recognition**.

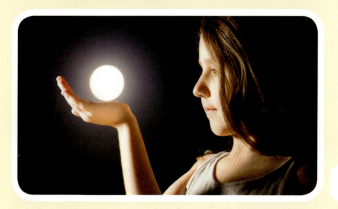

Talk about...

Why does a computer need to recognise images?

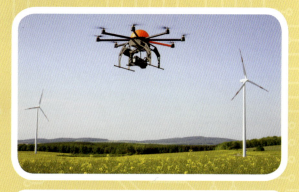

▲ This octocopter uses image recognition to work out if the crops are sick.

◄ Can a person really hold up the moon?

How does image recognition work?

The girl can ask questions to find out which shape the boy is holding.

→ How many sides does it have?

→ Is it a flat shape?

→ Is it a solid shape?

Can you think of any more questions?

2 This girl would like to know what shape the boy is holding.

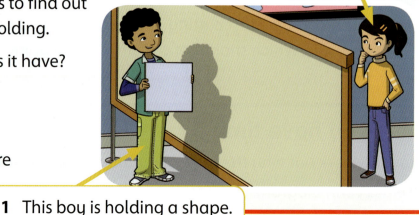

1 This boy is holding a shape.

94

A computer also uses shapes to recognise an image.

It makes the image into shapes by using 'edge detection'.

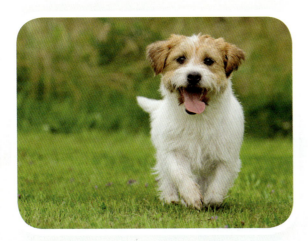 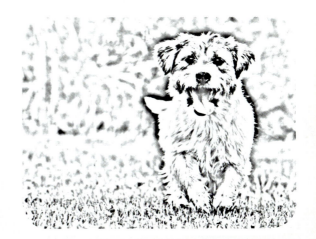

Then it compares what it detects to what it already knows.

This all happens very quickly.

Activity   Make your mosaic

Work in your group.

1 Continue making your small 'pixels' of colour for your mosaic.

2 Begin to stick the colours into the correct spaces on your large grid.

 If you have time…

1 Think about the human eye and brain. It takes a lot of work for a computer to recognise something. So can you imagine how complicated our eyes and brains are?

2 Imagine what it is like to be a blind person. How can a blind person recognise something that they cannot see?

You will learn:

➡ that digital images play an important role in society.

Look at these pictures.

This picture is of a wintery scene. Does this picture make you want to visit this place?

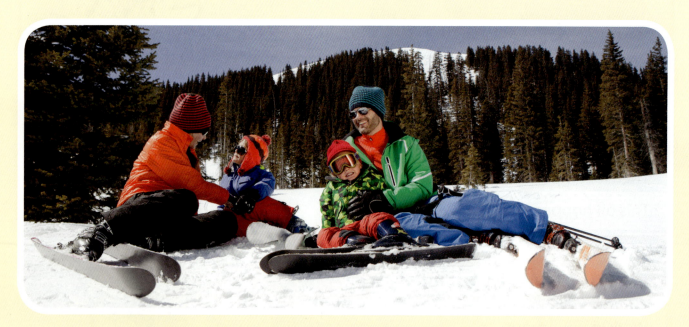

This is also a picture of a wintery scene, but it is very different.
How does it make you feel?

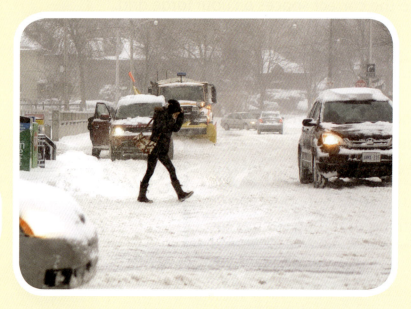

Talk about...

Look at all the pictures on these two pages. What words can you think of to describe these pictures?

Is it easy or difficult to think of words to describe them?

Images can make a difference to how people think and feel. This is because they:

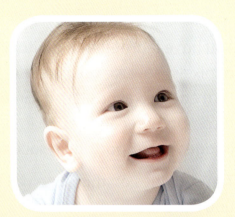

➜ show things that are important to us

➜ help us to remember things

➜ help us to see how other people live

➜ make us feel emotions like happiness, calm, sadness, sympathy and anger.

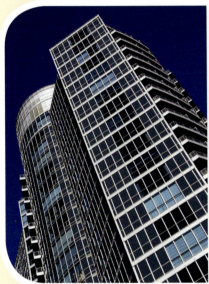 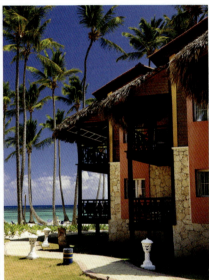 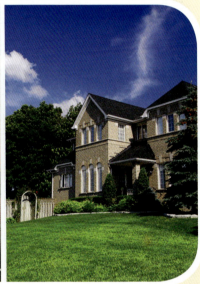

Because images are so powerful, we need to be responsible when we make images or share them with others.

It is quick and easy to take many digital images with mobile phones, digital cameras or tablet computers. When we take these images we need to think carefully about how to keep our images safe on the internet.

Activity Finish your mosaic

1 Work in your group to finish your mosaic.

2 Look at all the mosaics in the class. Can you see what is in each picture?

You have learned that digital images are made of pixels; how we use pixels to measure images; that each pixel has a Red, Green, Blue value; how a computer recognises an image; and why digital images are important in society.

The activities on this page will let you see how much you have learned.

1 Match the RGB values to the correct colour.

Colour		RGB value
Red	**a**	0, 0, 0
Green	**b**	255, 255, 255
Blue	**c**	0, 255, 0
Black	**d**	255, 0, 0
White	**e**	0, 0, 255
Yellow	**f**	255, 255, 0

2 How does a computer recognise an image?

_____

_____

Activity Image size

What is the size of this image?

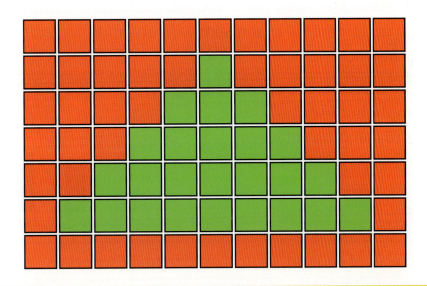

Activity Mixing colours

Is mixing RGB colours the same as mixing paint colours? Explain your answer to your teacher.

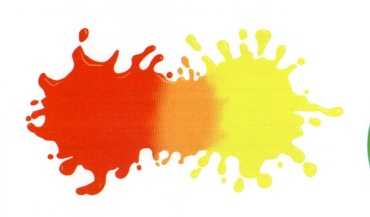

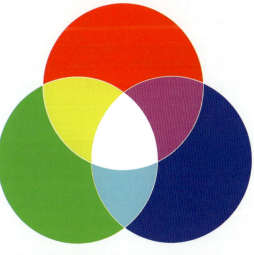

Glossary

align where your text goes on the page

animation a way of making the text or pictures on your slides move – you can make them appear or disappear in lots of different ways

attachment an additional file that is sent with an email, for example a picture or a document

bar chart a graph that uses rectangular bars to compare values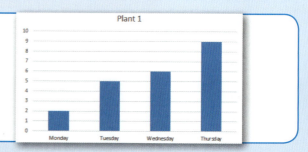

blocks small pieces of code, in *Scratch*, used to build scripts

callout an image label that consists of a text box with leader lines to parts of the image

cell reference the name of a cell – it is made of the column letter and the row number, for example C5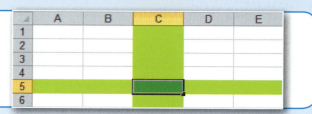

component a part of something

delete to remove or erase something

digital the way technology deals with data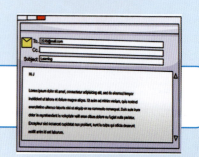

email written message that is shared electronically – short for 'electronic mail'

fixed loop a loop that repeats a fixed number of times

font the size, colour or style of your text

formula a calculation that generates a new value from data in the spreadsheet

hardware the physical objects that make up your computer

highlight to drag the cursor along a word or phrase to make it look highlighted

image a picture

import to add text or pictures from another place to your presentation, for example clip art or a picture you have made

insert to put text in

internet a global network of computers

key also called the legend – this gives the meaning of the colours or patterns used in the graph or chart

line graph a graph where points are connected by a continuous line – it is typically used to show a value that varies over time

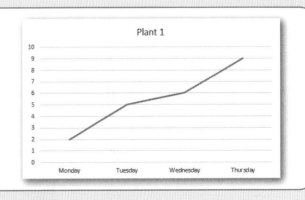

loop a script control that repeats the same commands over and over again

Glossary

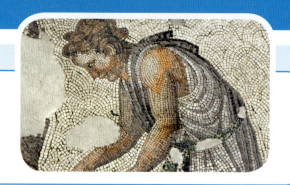

mosaic a picture made by putting together many small pieces of colour

output a result produced by a computer program

pharming emails that try to make you go to a website that is not real

phishing emails that try to get personal information about you

pixel a tiny dot of colour – pixel is short for 'picture element'

presentation an event you use to share ideas and information with an audience – you can use a slideshow to help make your presentation

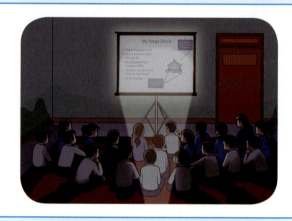

receive to get

recognition understanding what something is

resolution the number of pixels used to make an image

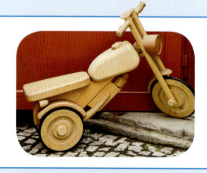
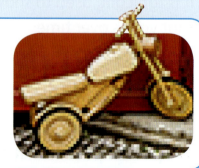

RGB value a number that tells us how much red, green and blue is in a pixel

0	51	102	153	204	255	255	255	0	0	0	255
0	51	102	153	204	255	0	0	0	255	255	255
0	51	102	153	204	255	0	255	255	255	0	0

right-click click with the right button of the mouse

Scratch a programming language for young people

script the area of the screen where you will create the program to control the sprite (in *Scratch*)

send to deliver to one or more recipient

shift key use this key to type the characters at the top of the keys

size how big or small something is

slide a part of your presentation – a presentation is made up of slides that show text and pictures

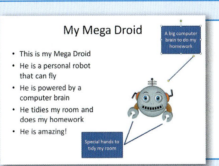

software the programs that makes your computer work

sort to reorganise a table of data into order, based on one of the columns of the table

spam a message you haven't asked for, and isn't important to you – spam often tries to sell you something or to cause problems on your computer

Glossary

spoofing emails sent from an email address that is not real

sprite an image on the screen that you control with a computer program

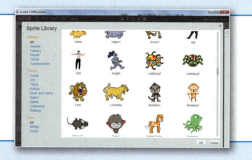

stage the area of the screen where you will see the sprite move (in *Scratch*)

store to save in a place that is safe and is easy to find again

style the way your text looks

symbol the characters on the key

transition a way of making the change between slides more interesting by using a pattern or movement

user the person who controls a computer program

user input values the user types while the program is running

value number data stored in a spreadsheet

virus protection software that prevents problems on your computer, and that finds and removes any problems

***x*-axis** the horizontal line at the bottom of a graph

***y*-axis** the vertical line to the left of a graph